Renal Diet Cookbook

Healthy Kidney Cookbook: Renal Diet Cookbook for Beginners Includes: Low Sodium, Low Potassium: Healthy Recipes to Avoid Dialysis

Chloe Health

Table of Contents

Introduction 6

Chapter One: The kidney 7

    Functions of the kidneys 8

    Chronic Kidney Disease 13

    Causes of Chronic Kidney Disease (CKD) 14

    Common symptoms of Chronic Kidney Disease 20

    Stages of Chronic Kidney Disease (CKD) 25

Chapter Two: Treatments for Kidney Failure (CKD) 28

    Dialysis 28

    Kidney Transplant 32

Chapter Three: Renal Diet 33

    Sodium 34

    Potassium 38

    Phosphorous 42

    Protein 45

    Fluid 45

Chapter Four: Kidney friendly Homemade Kitchen Staples and Seasonings 47

    Beef Stock 47

    Relish 50

    Vegetable Stock 52

    Chicken Stock 54

    Barbeque Sauce 56

Alfredo Sauce 58

Cinnamon Apple Sauce...60

Italian Seasoning 62

Breakfast 64

Blueberry Pancake.. 64

Vegetable Omelet...66

Pumpkin Pancake 68

Granola Breakfast Bowl...71

Simple Cumin Raisin Breakfast Quinoa 74

Blueberry Breakfast Smoothie Bowl 76

Blueberry Muffin 78

Overnight French toast...81

Cinnamon Bran Muffins 84

Corn Pudding 87

Breakfast Meatballs..90

Breakfast Frittata...93

Egg Sandwiches 96

Carrot Scramble...98

Eggplant Casserole 100

Meatloaf (no sauce) 103

Renal friendly Lunch, Dinner and Soups 105

Creamy Celery Soup 105

Cucumber Shrimp Soup..108

Ground beef Soup 110

Vegetable Soup 112

Pumpkin Chili 114

Rotisserie Chicken 117

Barley Soup 119

Chicken noodle soup 122

Chicken Rice Soup 124

Meatball Soup 127

Cauliflower Soup 130

Cabbage Stew 133

Cucumber Salad 136

Shrimp Scampi 138

Kidney Friendly Pizza 140

Irish stew 143

Turkey Stuffed Pepper 146

Orange Chicken 149

Indian Chickpea Curry (Chana Masala) 152

Tofu Stir Fry with Rice 155

Chicken Salad 158

Renal Friendly Snacks, Side Dishes, Desserts and Appetizers 160

Energy Balls 160

Roasted Chickpea Snack 162

Roasted Brussels sprouts and Bacon 164

Roasted Cauliflower Hummus 166

Keto Carrot Cake 169

Simple Roasted Butternut Squash 172

Blueberry Cookies 174

Macaroni Salad 177

Crispy Pork Belly 179

Cinnamon Protein Balls 182

Cream Cheese Cookies 184

Cinnamon Vanilla Shortbread 187

Chocolate Mug Cake 189

Tapioca Pudding 191

Black Bean Chocolate Brownies 193

Introduction

Overtime, chronic kidney disease has become a global issue. Every now and then we hear tragic stories of people that have chronic kidney disease. However, the big news here is that chronic kidney disease is not the end of the world. It can be managed and treated if discovered early. The best way to manage chronic kidney disease is to adopt a new way of eating. This kidney friendly way of eating is what we call the renal diet. With the renal diet, you can manage chronic kidney disease and avoid dialysis. Dialysis can be stressful and costly.

This book features awesome low sodium and low potassium recipes that are good for people who have chronic kidney disease. This book also contains important pieces of information about the kidneys, chronic kidney disease and renal diet.

Chapter one

The kidney

Since this book is all about kidney health, let's start my discussing the kidney and its importance to our body. The kidneys are two bean shaped fist-sized organs that can be found at the back of our abdominal cavity, just below the rib cage, on both sides of the spine. Our kidneys are so close to our back that it may be a bit difficult for a lay man to differentiate between back pain and kidney pain.

Physically, our kidneys are a bit small. Each kidney is about 4 to 5 inches long. But guess what! Their importance to the body system cannot be overemphasized. The kidneys perform important functions that are essential for the well being of the entire body. In fact, no human can survive if these functions are not executed. The kidneys are the body's filtration and waste management powerhouse. As such, if anyone suffers kidney failure, there is a need to find an alternative way to carry out the functions of the kidneys in the body if the person wants to survive. That brings us to the issue of dialysis, which shall be discussed later in this book. Those beans below your rib cage are not there for decoration!

So, if the kidneys are so important to our body system, what then is the job description of the kidneys in our body and why are the kidney functions indispensable to our body?

Functions of the kidneys

A. The kidneys filter the blood

At every point in time, the kidneys are busy filtering the blood in our body to get rid of waste and excess fluid in the body. On the average, your kidneys filters about 7.5 liters of blood per hour. Our kidneys house about a million filtering units that are medically referred to as "nephrons". Each of these nephrons is made up of glomerulus (a cluster of tiny blood vessels) and these tiny blood vessels are responsible for filtering blood in our body.

During the digestive process, your body absorbs the nutrients in the foods you eat. Afterwards, the absorbed nutrients are used to feed your cells and repair your cells. Absorbed nutrients are also converted to energy to power your brain. Once your body has utilized the amount of nutrients needed at a point in time, excess nutrients are released into the blood as waste products. Urea, salt and creatinine constitute a larger percentage of these waste products. The problem here is that waste products released into the blood can build up and become toxic overtime if not discarded. This is where the kidneys come in to rescue the body from the danger of allowing waste products to build up in the blood stream.

As the heart is pumping oxygen filled blood to all parts of the body, blood with wastes flows into our kidneys through the renal arteries. As the blood flows into our kidney, it is distributed into the nephrons, where it is filtered by a cluster of tiny blood vessels called glomerulus. The glomeruli have the capacity to filter out the waste in the blood. Each glomerulus is so tiny that only smaller molecules can pass through it. These smaller molecules constitute the waste products in our blood. As such, when our blood is filtered by the glomeruli, the smaller molecules are allowed to flow into the tubules as waste while larger molecules which include protein and red blood cells are retained. After filtration, filtered blood, containing protein and red blood cells is released back into our body system through the renal veins. The waste products will eventually be transported into the bladder through the ureters as urine.

This is how the kidney filters our blood everyday to avoid the buildup of toxic waste in the bloodstream. If your kidneys fail, waste products will start building up in your body. This can lead to a lot of crisis medically and eventually lead to death. I like to compare the importance of kidneys, as the ultimate blood filters, to the body to that of a fuel filter to a car engine. If car's fuel filter is bad, the engine will get clogged up with dirt and it may eventually stop working if the issue is not attended to. Likewise, if anyone suffers kidney failure, their blood will get clogged up with toxins and this may lead to a lot of negative health issues or death if not attended to immediately.

B. The kidneys regulate your body water/fluid

The kidneys play the most significant role in balancing the water content in our body. Our body's water content needs to be balanced as excess body fluid or insufficient body fluid can cause problems in our body system. This function of the kidneys can be described in two different situations.

On the one hand, when the water content in our body is excess, the kidneys perform a significant role in ensuring that excess water is removed from the blood and excreted to keep our body fluid balanced.

How is this done?

The excretion of excess water from our body takes a cause and effect format, one state stimulating the occurrence of other activities in the body. When we consume excess water, it will dilute our blood and increase the volume of blood in the body. Once the volume of blood increases, the hydrostatic pressure of our blood will rise above normal. Consequently, our kidneys will respond to this by increasing ultrafiltration – the filtration of blood by the glomeruli. With increased ultrafiltration, the rate at which the glomeruli filter the blood will increase, thereby enhancing the prompt removal of excess water from the blood. During the filtration process, excess water will be transported to the bladder through the ureters to form urine. In cases like this, the urine content is usually diluted and less yellowish. So, whenever you go into the toilet to pass out a lot of diluted urine content, it means that your kidneys have worked hard to get rid of excess fluid from your blood.

On the other hand, the kidneys are also saddled with the responsibility of increasing our body's fluid content when the body is dehydrated. This is normally achieved through the process of reabsorption. The kidneys in conjunction with the hypothalamus perform a significant role in balancing body fluid during dehydration. Our body loses water every day through urine, sweat, breathing and even evaporation of water from the skin, especially during sunny days. Thus, it is important for us to drink enough water every day to replenish lost water content. But if you do not drink enough water at a point in time, you may be dehydrated.

During dehydration, your blood plasma will become thicker because it contains less water content. Once this happens, it will trigger some activities in your body system. These activities will start from the hypothalamus - a small region of our brain located at the base of the brain, near the pituitary gland. The hypothalamus, through the posterior pituitary gland, will release a hormone called the antidiuretic hormone (ADH) into the body system. This hormone will then send a signal to the kidney to reabsorb water from urine in order to dilute blood plasma. In response to this signal, the nephron in the kidney will start reabsorbing water and solute from the waste in the tubules. Reabsorbed water will then be released into the blood to dilute the blood plasma. This process is responsible for the formation of concentrated yellowish urine.

The foregoing processes explain how the kidney regulates our body fluid content. I guess you now see one more reason why the kidneys are so important to our body system.

C. The kidneys aid the creation of red blood cells in our body

The kidneys also play a vital role in preventing anemia by aiding the production of red blood cells in our body. Healthy kidneys are responsible for the production of a hormone called erythropoietin (EPO). EPO is essential for the production of red blood cells in our body. The function of the red blood cells is to circulate oxygen to body organs and tissues so that they can function properly. This means that a reduction in the amount of red blood cells in our body will result in to a reduction in the supply of oxygen in our body, thereby reducing the effectiveness of body organs and tissues in our body. Anytime the kidney senses a reduction in body oxygen, it will produce erythropoietin (EPO). EPO will then stimulate our bone marrows to produce more red blood cells in other to increase body oxygen circulation and regulate the function of body organs and tissue. The parts of our kidney that produce EPO are called the juxtaglomerular cells – cells that are close to the glomerulus.

D. The kidneys regulate blood pressure

Apart from the fact that the kidneys regulate blood pressure by getting rid of excess blood fluid, the kidneys also contribute to the regulation of blood pressure by regulating blood potassium level, regulating blood sodium level and also producing renin – a hormone which is essential for regulating blood pressure.

Sodium and potassium are two electrolytes that have a major effect on our blood pressure level. Sodium is responsible for increasing blood pressure and potassium is responsible for reducing blood pressure. If blood sodium is too low or the blood potassium is too high, it will lead to low blood pressure. Likewise, if blood sodium is too high or blood potassium is too low, blood pressure will rise. It is the job of our kidneys to keep our blood sodium level and potassium level balanced in order to regulate blood pressure.

Whenever the kidneys sense an abnormal reduction in blood pressure, the kidneys will produce and release renin into the blood stream. Renin will then convert angiotensinogen (a precursor protein that is primarily produced and released by the liver) into angiotensin 1. Subsequently, angiotensin 1 will be converted to angiotensin 2 in the lungs by an enzyme called Angiotensin-Converting Enzyme (ACE). Once angiotensin 2 is formed it will constrict the blood vessels in our body, thereby causing blood pressure to increase.

Angiotensins 2 will also stimulate the production of another hormone called aldostrone in the adrenal gland. When aldostrone is released, it will stimulate the renal tubules to increase the reabsorption of sodium and water into the blood stream and increase the excretion of potassium from the blood. This action will also increase blood pressure.

E. The kidneys promote bone health

Our kidneys are essential for maintaining healthy bones because they actively regulate the level of calcium and phosphorus in our body.

The kidneys aid bone health by activating vitamin D. The foods will consume contain an inactive form of vitamin D, which is usually activated by the kidney. When the kidney activates vitamin D, it is converted into calcitriol which facilitates the absorption of calcium by our intestine and indirectly improve bone health. Without calcitriol, our intestine cannot absorb calcium and the inability of the intestine to absorb calcium will lead to bone weakness. Calcitriol helps the kidneys to maintain blood calcium and improve bone health.

The kidneys also aid bone health by getting rid of excess phosphorous in our body. Although our body needs phosphorous to form and repair our bones and teeth, excess blood phosphorous can extract calcium from our bones and cause bone weakness. To avoid this, the kidneys are needed to filter out excess blood phosphorus into the urinary tubules during filtration.

Chronic Kidney Disease

Having discussed the functions and importance of the kidneys, let us talk about Chronic Kidney Disease (CKD), causes of chronic kidney diseases and the symptoms of chronic kidney disease. Kidney disease is a condition where the kidneys can no longer perform their functions effectively. Kidney disease is not spontaneous; it happens gradually and in stages. In fact, people with kidney disease may not notice that they have kidney disease until kidney functions have reduced immensely. Kidney disease is chronic; that is, it cannot be cured. However, it can be treated or managed, particularly in the early stages of the disease. If kidney disease is not treated immediately, it will lead to kidney failure. And when that happens, the only way the patient can survive is through dialysis or kidney transplant. We shall talk about dialysis and kidney transplant in this book later. And remember, the purpose of this book is to help chronic kidney disease patients to avoid dialysis/ kidney transplant. Now, let us look into the causes of Chronic Kidney Disease (CKD).

Causes of Chronic Kidney Disease (CKD)
A. Diabetes

Uncontrolled diabetes has been reported to be the leading cause of kidney disease. A lot of medical studies have proved that diabetes patients are at high risk of chronic kidney disease (CKD). Diabetes is another chronic disease that causes an abnormal increase in blood sugar. Abnormal increase in blood sugar will increase the level of waste product in our blood, thereby giving the kidney more work to do. If this continues uncontrolled over time, the glomerulus will worn out and start to leak as a result of constant excess work. This will result to a decrease in the effectiveness of the kidney as the glomerulus would have expanded and they would not be able to retain blood proteins anymore. Thus, protein contents that should be retained in the blood will now be released into the tubules and excreted as urine. This is the reason for the presence of protein in the urine of chronic kidney disease (CKD) patients. It is advisable for diabetes patients to go for kidney disease test to be sure that their kidneys are healthy.

B. High blood pressure

High blood pressure ranks as the second leading cause of chronic kidney disease (CKD). Blood pressure is the force by which blood flows through our body. When blood pressure is high, it will start to strain the blood vessels in the body. If this condition continues uncontrolled over time, it will damage body blood vessels, including the ones in the kidney. Once the glomeruli (tiny blood vessels in the kidneys) are damaged, their blood filtration rate will start to decrease gradually until they are unable to filter blood again. The inability of the kidney to filter blood is called kidney failure- the last stage of chronic kidney diseases. If you have high blood pressure, you have to take necessary measures to regulate your blood pressure and also go for a kidney disease test to ensure that your kidneys are healthy. Chronic kidney disease is best treated and managed when it is discovered early.

C. Glomerulonephritis

This is another leading cause of kidney disease. Glomerulonephritis is a disease that affects our glomerulus. It causes an abnormal inflammation of the glomerulus, thereby reducing the effectiveness of the glomerulus. If this condition persists over time, it can lead to kidney failure. There are two types of glomerulonephritis: (i) acute glomerulonephritis and (ii) chronic glomerulonephrtis. Acute glomerulonephritis happens suddenly and it is usually triggered by the effect of other diseases such as strep throat infection, lupus, good pasture syndrome and polyarteritis. Chronic glomerulonephritis on the other hand is usually hereditary. The symptoms of glomerulonephritis include:

      I. Blood urine
      II. Swelling in the ankles and face
      III. Urinating less often
      IV. Puffiness of the face, especially in the morning
      V. Foamy urine
      VI. High blood pressure
      VII. Nosebleeds
      VIII. Abdominal pain
      IX. Urinating frequently at nighttime

It is highly important for you to visit your doctor for check up immediately if you notice any of these symptoms. Untreated glomerulonephritis will cause irreversible damage to your kidneys and can lead to kidney failure. It is advisable for people who have history of chronic glomerulonephritis in their family to go for check up periodically to ensure good kidney health.

D. Polycystic kidney disease (PKD)

Polycystic kidney disease, just like chronic glomerulonephritis, is genetic. People who have polycystic kidney disease (PKD) inherited it from one of their parents or both. Polycystic kidney disease causes a cluster of cysts (noncancerous fluid filled sac-like bumps that can develop in any part of the body) to develop in the kidney. Development of cyst in the kidneys will make the kidneys swell abnormally and reduce their effectiveness. If this condition is not managed properly, it can lead to kidney failure. Common symptoms of polycystic kidney disease include:

      i. Joint pain
      ii. Abdominal pain

    iii. Fatigue
    iv. Nail abnormalities
    v. Kidney stones
    vi. Constant back pain
    vii. Pain in the kidney area (your back and loin, just below the rib cage)
    viii. Bruises
    ix. Blood in urine

E. Kidney stones

Kidney stones, also known as nephrolithiasis, can also cause chronic kidney disease (CKD) and lead to kidney failure if it is not treated on time. Kidney stones are crystal-like mineral formations that can develop in the kidneys, bladder, ureters as well as in the urethra. Kidney stones usually develop when your urine is too concentrated. Some of the concentrated minerals or waste products in the urine may start to stick together, forming kidney stones. Concentrated urine can be prompted by dehydration, inflammatory bowel disease, persistent consumption of excess salt, protein or glucose, renal tubular acidosis, obesity, chronic diarrhea, hyparathyrodism and some other medical conditions. Some types of kidney stone disease are also hereditary. Calcium formed kidney stones are the most common type of kidney stone. Kidney stones can also be formed by uric acid, cystine, xanthine and phosphate. The easiest way to prevent kidney stones is by drinking enough water every day. You should drink about 10 glasses of water or more every day. This will help to dilute your urine and prevent the formation of concentrated urine.

People with kidney stones are at higher risk of chronic kidney disease (CKD) Kidney stones, especially the ones that are not too big, can eventually be passed out as urine but some of them can get to obstruct some tracts in the kidney and trigger kidney disease. Common symptoms of kidney stones include:

    I. Blood urine
    II. Painful urination
    III. Smelling urine
    IV. Pain in the kidney area (your side and back, below your rib cage)
    V. Nausea and vomiting
    VI. Pain in the lower abdominal area
    VII. Fever and chills

If you sense one or more of these symptoms, you should visit your doctor immediately for check up. People whose family has a history of kidney stone should also go for check up periodically to be sure that their kidneys are free from stones.

F. Kidney Trauma

This is when parts of our kidneys are damaged as a result of an external force. There are two types of kidney trauma: blunt kidney trauma and penetrating trauma. Blunt trauma is usually caused by, car accident, fall or assault while penetrating trauma results from gunshot or stabbing. Kidney trauma can trigger chronic kidney disease. In fact, kidney trauma, especially penetrating, trauma can lead to acute kidney failure if it is not treated immediately. The kidneys of patients who are victims of severe back injury, abdominal injury, rib fractures, car accident, gunshot, stabbing and assault should be examined immediately. Symptoms of kidney trauma include:

    I. Hematura - blood in the urine
    II. Skin bruising
    III. Skin discoloration

IV. Low blood pressure
V. Pain in the kidney area (your back and sides, below the rib cage)
VI. Anemia

No form of kidney trauma is minor; kidney injury sustained during trauma can pave way for chronic kidney disease as well as acute kidney failure. If you are a victim of car accident, assault, gunshot or stabbing, visit a doctor immediately. Our kidneys happen to be one of those body organs that are very susceptible to injury during accidents.

G. Drugs and toxins

A number of chronic kidney disease cases stem from the adverse effects of some drugs on our renal system. More people are now fond of misusing drugs due to the increase in the production of different drugs and the easy accessibility to these drugs. Self medication has become the order of the day; people just go to the counter to buy drugs without prescription. This has lead to an increase in cases of chronic kidney disease because our kidneys are quite susceptible to the adverse effects of drug abuse. Our kidneys are at the receiving end here because they are saddled with the responsibility of removing the excess toxins released into the blood as a result of improper drug usage.

Such drugs include antibiotics; non steroidal anti inflammatory drugs (NSAID) such as ibuprofen and aspirin; laxatives; supplements; diuretics and aminoglycosides (AMG). I do not think we really need to give a long list of all these drugs. The bottom line here is that you should stay away from using drugs without prescription. And if you have been abusing the use of any of the listed drugs or other drugs, please visit your doctor to check if your kidneys have not been affected.

H. Smoking

Smokers are at high risk of chronic kidney disease (CKD) and kidney cancer. Smoking can affect the kidneys in a lot of ways, directly and indirectly. To start with, smoking can affect your kidney health indirectly because it can trigger high blood pressure, which is a leading cause of kidney disease. Smoking also tightens blood vessels in the body. This usually results into slow flow of blood and oxygen to the body organs, including the kidneys. The kidneys, just like all body organs, need blood and oxygen to function properly; thus, their effectiveness will reduce when they are not getting enough blood and oxygen. This can eventually trigger chronic kidney disease (CKD).

More so, nicotine, one of the components of a cigarette, can facilitate the progression of damage in kidney disease patients. As such, patients of chronic kidney disease as well as people with healthy kidneys should stay away from smoking. Abstaining from smoking can be a little bit difficult because of the addictive effect of nicotine, but if you really want your kidneys to be healthy or you want to avoid dialysis, you need to stop smoking now.

Common symptoms of Chronic Kidney Disease

One funny thing about chronic kidney disease is that people who have the disease do not normally sense the symptoms during the early stage of the disease. Most people get to sense the symptoms when the effectiveness of the kidneys has decreased greatly. And even when some of the symptoms are noticed, some people do not recognize these symptoms or pay attention to them. In fact, some people may not know that they have chronic kidney disease (CKD) until their kidney fails. So, do not be surprised when you are told that your neighbor who played table tennis with you a day before collapsed on the next day while cooking as a result of critical kidney condition. Let us quickly look into some of the symptoms of chronic kidney disease (CKD).

A. Anemia induced fatigue

Anemia is a negative health condition that has to do with the insufficiency of red blood cells in the body. The red blood cells transport blood and oxygen to all organs and tissues of the body. Body organs need the oxygen circulated by red blood cells to function effectively. As hinted earlier, a kidney secreted hormone, Erithropoetin (EPO), is essential in the production of more red blood cells in the body. When you have chronic kidney disease (CKD) your kidneys may stop producing enough EPO. This will in turn affect the availability of enough red blood cells in the body. In this light, your body organs, including the brain, will not be getting enough oxygen. This will cause weakness in your body organs and lid to fatigue.

B. Memory loss or inability to concentrate

This symptom comes with anemia. It is as a result of insufficient supply of oxygen to the brain.

C. Bone weakness

When the kidneys are damaged, they may not be able maintain the balance of calcium and phosphorus in the body. Thus, your bones will start getting weak.

On the one hand, your blood calcium level will decrease. Calcitrol, the active form of vitamin D which is usually activated by the kidney, is responsible for the absorption of calcium by the intestines. When your kidneys are not at their best, there may be a reduction in the production of calcitrol. This will reduce the absorption of calcium from foods and decrease blood calcium level. Thus, your bones may start to weaken as your bones need enough calcium to stay healthy.

On the other hand, chronic kidney disease can lead to the availability of too much phosphorus in the blood. Unhealthy kidneys will not be able to filter out excess phosphorus from the blood. Excess phosphorus is quite inimical to your bone health. Although phosphorus is essential for bone health, excess phosphorus will extract calcium from the bones and cause bone weakness.

D. Foamy urine

When the glomerulus in your kidneys are no longer effective, protein contents that should be retained in the blood will be escaping into the tubules to form urine. The presence of protein in your urine will cause your urine to foam. Foamy urine is a common symptom of chronic disease. Unfortunately, most people do not pay attention to their urine when they urinate.

E. Swelling legs, feet and ankles / puffy eyes

Chronic Kidney disease causes toxins and excess mineral to start building up in the blood as the kidneys will be unable to get rid of these waste products. Over time, these toxins and excess mineral will start lodging in your legs, feet, ankle, joints and face. If you notice any abnormal swelling in one or more of these areas, visit your doctor immediately. Chronic kidney disease (CKD) is best managed when it is discovered early.

F. Constant back pain

This is one symptom of chronic kidney disease (CKD) that people don't take seriously. I guess we all see back pain as a normal thing. Chronic kidney disease can cause constant pain in your lower back area, below the rib cage. If you notice constant pain in your groin or lower back area, you should visit your doctor for check up. Pain relief drugs may not help things here.

G. High blood pressure

Unhealthy kidneys are unable to regulate blood fluid level. This allows minerals like sodium to build up in the body. The presence of excess fluid and sodium in the blood stream will increase your blood pressure level. Another bad news here is that increased blood pressure can cause more damage to the kidneys. Remember, high blood pressure is the second leading cause of kidney disease. As such, it is very important for high blood patients to take kidney disease tests periodically.

H. Nausea and vomiting

The presence of excessive fluid in the blood stream as a result of chronic kidney disease can make you nauseate and vomit. Though nauseating and vomiting are symptoms of different health conditions, it is advisable to always visit a doctor to know the cause of it. Don't just go to the chemist to get drugs; visit a doctor to know the true cause of the nausea and vomiting.

I. Dry and Itchy skin

The buildup of excessive fluid, especially phosphorus, in the blood can cause your skin to itch. Excessive build up of urea on the blood can also cause your skin to be dry. Itchy skin also comes with anemia, which is one of the complications of chronic kidney disease. Cases of dry itchy skin should be given prompt medical attention.

J. Loss of appetite and abnormal changes in food taste

Excessive blood fluid can also affect your taste bud. Foods will start tasting metallic to you and you may start losing appetite.

K. Shortness of breath

When excess fluid starts building up in your blood as a result of unhealthy kidneys, they will start lodging in your body organs including the lungs. The presence of excess fluid in the lungs can cause shortness of breath. Cases of shortness of breath should be given prompt attention medically. Put yourself together and go for a checkup.

L. Bad breath

People with chronic kidney disease can have bad breath as a result of the deposit of excess fluid and electrolytes in the blood and body organs.

M. Feeling cold always

The buildup of excess fluid and minerals in the blood can pave way for hypothermia - a state where the body temperature drops abnormally. Kidney disease patient may also feel cold always as a result of limited red blood cells in their body.

N. Muscle cramp

Frequent muscle cramps, especially leg cramp, are also a symptom of chronic kidney disease (CKD). High blood pressure, a common symptom of chronic kidney disease (CKD), can stretch and narrow the blood vessels in legs. This may cause frequent leg cramps in people who have chronic kidney disease. Frequent muscle cramps can also be triggered by the presence of excess fluid and electrolytes in the blood. If you have been having frequent muscle cramps, especially leg cramps, visit a doctor for check up.

If you notice one or more of these highlighted symptoms of chronic kidney disease (CKD), do not hesitate to visit your doctor for proper check up.

Stages of Chronic Kidney Disease (CKD)

Chronic kidney disease (CKD) is not a sudden condition; it occurs in stages. Patients move from one stage of chronic kidney disease to the other as the effectiveness of the kidneys decreases over time until they get to the last stage. The last stage of chronic kidney disease is kidney failure. At this stage, patients need dialysis or kidney transplant to survive.

Stages of chronic kidney disease are identified according to a patient's estimated Glomerular Filtration Rate (GFR) - the rate at which the kidney filters toxins from the blood. GFR is considered the yardstick for measuring overall kidney functions.GFR is usually determined by examining the level of blood creatinine, a waste product that is produced during muscle metabolism, in conjunction with other factors such as age, sex, body size and race. . Let us highlight the stages of chronic kidney disease (CKD).

Stage 1

At stage one, the functions of the kidneys are still normal and patients may not notice any obvious symptoms. But protein can be noticed in patients' urine if tested. The estimated glomerular filtration rate (GFR) of the kidneys at stage one is 90 ml per minute or above. This is similar to GFR of a healthy kidney.

Stage 2

Stage two chronic kidney disease (CKD) characterizes a mild decrease in kidney functions. At this point, a little rise in the level of creatinine in the blood can be noticed if the patient is tested. The estimated glomerular filtration rate (GFR) of the kidney in stage two is around 60 to 89 ml per minute.

Stage 3

Stage 3 is often referred to as the middle stage of chronic kidney disease (CKD). It is the most common category of chronic kidney disease. At stage 3 there is a moderate decrease in kidney functions and patients must have started to sense some complications of chronic kidney disease. These complications include anemia, high blood pressure, bone weakness and fatigue. The third stage of chronic kidney disease (CKD) occurs in two phases. The estimated glomerular filtration rate (GFR) for phase one stage 3 of CKD is around 45 to 59 ml per minutes while phase two features an estimated GFR of 30 to 44 ml per minute.

Stage 4

At stage four, the functions of the kidney will have decreased immensely and the patient will be faced with a lot of negative health conditions associated with chronic kidney disease (CKD). This stage is associated with severity. At this stage, doctors will already be planning for dialysis or kidney transplant. The estimated glomerular filtration rate (GFR) in stage four is around 15 to 29 ml per minute.

Stage 5

Stage five is the last stage of chronic kidney disease. This is the stage where the kidneys finally fail. The estimated glomerular filtration rate (GFR) is below 15 ml per minutes. The kidneys may still be able to function a bit but the level of the kidney functions at this stage will not be enough to keep the patient alive. At stage five the patient will need dialysis or kidney transplant to survive.

Chapter Two

Treatments for Kidney Failure (CKD)

There are two treatments for chronic kidney disease (CKD): dialysis and kidney transplant.

Dialysis

The main purpose of this book is to help chronic kidney disease patients to maintain the condition in order to avoid dialysis. Thus, it is important that we talk about dialysis. Dialysis, also known as kidney replacement therapy, is a process of getting rid of waste products, toxins, excess fluid and electrolytes from the blood of kidney failure patients. Dialysis gives hope to people whose kidneys have failed. There are two main types of dialysis: Hemodialysis and peritoneal dialysis.

    A. Hemodialysis

Hemodialysis is a type of dialysis that is performed with the use of a dialysis machine. Blood will be passed into the machine via a tube connected to an "access" (we shall talk about "access" later under this subtopic). The machine will then filter the blood to get rid of excess fluid and waste product from the blood. There is a part of the dialysis machine called the dialyzer. The dialyzer acts a filter during hemodialysis. It is modeled after the glomeruli. The dialyzer ensures that toxins and waste products are filtered out of the blood while protein and red blood cells, which are too big to escape the filter, are retained. After filtration, clean blood containing protein and red blood cells will then be released into the blood via another tube. Patients usually undergo hemodialysis thrice in a week and each hemodialysis session can last up to four hours or more depending on the amount of waste in the blood and the capacity of the dialysis machine. Hemodialysis is the most preferred dialysis treatment to most kidney failure patients.

What is an access?

When chronic kidney disease (CKD) gets to the fourth stage in a patient, doctors will start preparing for dialysis or kidney transplant. If the chosen kidney failure treatment is hemodialysis, preparation includes creating a point in the body where blood can be accessed for hemodialysis. Access creation involves minor surgical operation. An access is created to ensure easy and fast flow of blood into the dialysis machine during hemodialysis. There are two main types of access: Fistula and graft

Fistula

To create a fistula, a doctor will join an artery and vein together in your arm (forearm or upper arm), under the skin to create a bigger blood vessel. A fistula is usually created few months to the commencement of dialysis so that the created blood vessel must have healed before then. During hemodialysis, two needles connected to two different tubes will be inserted into the fistula, one passing blood into the dialysis machine and the other releasing clean blood into the body.

Graft

A graft serves as a substitute to fistula in cases where the patient's blood vessels cannot be used to create a fistula. A graft is usually created by using a special soft tube to connect an artery and vein together, under the skin. A graft takes about four to six weeks to heal completely before they can be used for dialysis.

B. Peritoneal Dialysis

Peritoneal dialysis serves as an alternative to hemodialysis. Peritoneal dialysis is not entirely artificial; this type of dialysis makes use of the peritoneum as a dialyzer to filter the blood of the patient. The peritoneum is a serous membrane which lines and covers the abdominal cavity and the abdominal organs. This membrane acts as a natural filter through which waste is extracted from the blood during peritoneal dialysis.

How does peritoneal dialysis work?

Before the commencement of peritoneal dialysis, the patient needs to undergo a minor surgery in order to insert a permanent catheter into the patient's abdomen. The surgery will take a few weeks to heal before the catheter can be used for peritoneal dialysis.

During peritoneal dialysis, a cleansing fluid called dialysate will be released into a patient's abdomen through the catheter. Dialysate help to absorb waste products such as creatinine and urea from the blood flowing through the abdominal lining. The peritoneum allows waste to be released into the dialysate fluid while it retains useful blood contents such as red blood cells and protein. The dialysate will be allowed to stay in the abdomen for a specific time frame, about two hours or more. The specified time the dialysate spends in the patient's abdomen is refered to as the dwell time. After the dwell time, the dialysate which must have absorbed blood waste will be drain out of the stomach into a waste bag through the catheter. The bag to which the dialysate is drained is called the drainage bag. The drainage is to be removed and discarded after each dialysis. Peritoneal dialysis is quite simple to perform; it is usually done by the patients and it can be performed at work, at home or while traveling.

There are two types of peritoneal dialysis:

I. Continual Ambulatory Peritoneal Dialysis (CAPD)
II. Continuous Circling Peritoneal Dialysis (CCPD)

I. **Continuous Ambulatory Peritoneal Dialysis (CAPD)**

This form of peritoneal dialysis is usually performed manually, without the aid of any machine. The patient will first have to fill his or her abdomen with a bag of dialysate solution and later drain out the solution after the dwell time. The filling and draining system in continuous ambulatory peritoneal dialysis relies on gravity. The patient has to repeat the process three to four times daily with a new drainage bag and a new dialysate bag. The process of filling and draining dialysate solution from the abdomen in peritoneal dialysis is called exchange.

II. **Continuous Circling Peritoneal Dialysis (CCPD)**

This form of peritoneal dialysis is usually performed while the patient is sleeping with the aid of a machine known as the cycler. CCPD is also known as Automatic Peritoneal Dialysis (APD). All the patient has to do is to connect the cycler to the catheter before going to bed at night. While the patient is sleeping, the cycler will perform about 3 to 5 exchanges automatically. At each exchange, the cycle will fill the abdomen with dialysate and wait for the dwell time before draining the solution into a sterile bag. The sterile bag will be discarded by the patient in the morning. CCPD requires the patient to be connected to the cycler for about 10 to 12 hours every night. It means if you are the type that doesn't stay long in bed; you may have to adjust your sleeping habit to facilitate effective CCPD.

After the night's dialysis, the patient may need to carry out one manual exchange whose dwell time lasts the whole day. That is, you will allow the dialysate to remain in yourabdomen while you are out, doing your things during the day.

Kidney Transplant

Kidney transplant is another treatment for kidney failure. Kidney transplantation is a surgical operation performed to place a healthy kidney, removed from a donor, into a kidney failure patient. One amazing thing is that our body can function well with just one kidney. So, when a person's kidneys fail, another person can offer to donate one of their healthy kidneys to the kidney failure patient. After the kidney transplant, the patient and the donor can now live a healthy life with one healthy kidney each. In some cases, the donor may be deceased; healthy kidneys can be removed from someone who just died to replace that of a kidney failure patient. Thus, we have two categories of kidney transplantation: living-donor kidney transplantation and deceased donor kidney transplantation. Living donors are usually close relatives of the patient. To receive a healthy kidney from a deceased donor, you have to be on a national waiting list. The procedures for benefiting from deceased donor transplantation may vary across countries.

Chapter Three

Renal Diet

Chronic kidney disease (CKD) cannot be cured as damages to parts of our kidneys are usually irreversible. However, the good news is that you can slow down the progression of the disease into critical stages by embracing a new lifestyle and way of eating. The kind of foods we eat indubitably has a great effect on the health of our body organs, including the kidneys. As a chronic kidney disease patient, the best thing to do is to switch to a kidney friendly diet. This kind of diet is popular known as the renal diet.

Although chronic kidney disease cannot be cured, the renal diet can help chronic kidney disease (CKD) patients to retain kidney functions and delay kidney failure for years. The major effect of the renal diet on our kidneys is that it reduces the workload of the kidney, thereby making them to last longer.

How is this achieved?

A proper renal diet is geared towards reducing the amount of sodium, phosphorus, potassium, protein and fluid consumed by a chronic kidney disease (CKD) patient. When this is achieved, the level of waste released into the blood after the body has extracted the useful materials in the food we eat will reduce. Consequently, the kidney will be relieved as they now have fewer waste products to filter. It would not cost the glomerulus much stress to filter the blood when the level of waste in the blood is low. Now, let us talk about how and why a chronic kidney disease (CKD) patient should regulate their intake of sodium, potassium, protein and phosphorus.

Sodium

Sodium is one of the essential electrolytes needed by our body. Sodium helps in regulating our blood pressure, balancing the level of water in our cells, facilitating proper muscle and nerves function and regulating the acid-base level of the blood.

Healthy kidneys get rid of excess sodium in our blood. However, damaged kidneys will not be to excrete excess blood sodium. This will result in the buildup of sodium in the blood. The consumption of excess sodium can negatively affect the kidneys of a chronic kidney disease patient in two ways. First, it will increase the workload of the damaged kidneys, thus causing more damages. Secondly, excess sodium will start to build up in the blood as a result of the kidneys inability to get rid of it. The buildup of excess sodium in the blood will lead to high blood pressure, a condition that can accelerate the progression of chronic kidney disease into critical stages and cause kidney failure.

As such, you have to watch the amount of sodium you consume per day. Try to limit your sodium consumption to 140 – 150 milligrams per serving for snacks and 400 – 500 mg per serving for meals. Generally, chronic kidney disease (CKD) patients are advised to keep their daily intake of sodium between 1500 to 2000 milligrams. However, you may need to consult a kidney dietitian to be sure of the right amount of sodium you are allowed to consume per day, depending on the condition of your kidneys and other variables.

How to control your sodium intake

1. Stay away from food containing high sodium:

When we talk about sodium consumption, some people think it's all about table salt, sea salt or other forms of salt. The fact is that some of the foods you eat are high in sodium even before you season them with salt. In fact, about 75% of the sodium we consume comes from the foods we eat, without added salt. Below is a list of foods containing high sodium:

Processed meats and fish

Smoked, canned, salted, picked or cure meats such as ham, bacon, pepperoni, regular canned salmon and tuna, sausage, wieners, deli meats, corn beef, salami, cold cuts, pepperoni, flakes of chicken, flakes of turkey, flakes of ham, potted meat, salted dried fish, salted smoked fish, salted fish, hot dogs, kosher meats, devilled ham, luncheon meat and so on.

Salt and salt seasonings

Salted mixed spices, seasoned pepper, lemon pepper, garlic salt, pink salt, seasoning salt, table salt, kosher salt, sea salt, bouillon cubes, flavor enhancers, onion salt, celery salt, lite salt, steak spice and so on.

Sauces

Soy sauce, barbeque sauce, teriyaki sauce, salted tomato sauce, tartar sauce, Worcestershire sauce, tobacco sauce, steak sauce, salted tomato sauce, Taco sauce, picante sauce, oyster sauce, chili sauce.

Condiments

Monosodium glutamate (MSG), salsa, meat tenderizers, ketchup, sauerkraut, salad dressing, olives, pickles and relish.

Canned foods

Salted canned soups, salted canned vegetables, canned juices, canned broths

Snacks

Salted snacks such as chips, pretzels, popcorn, cheezies, peanuts, salted crackers, pork rinds, salted nuts and so on.

Dairy and milk products

Butter milk, feta cheese, blue cheese, sweetened condensed milk, malted milk, processed cheese, Parmesan cheese, commercial milk drinks and so on.

Other high sodium foods include baking soda, baking powder, cheese bread, cookies, bacon fat, ovaltine, cream of tartar, corn syrup, salted butter, cheese bread, waffles, meat patties, instant potatoes, scalloped potato mix, salted margarine, salted mayonnaise, salted gravy and so on.

2. Pay attention to food nutritional fact labels

The list of both high sodium foods and low sodium foods is endless; you cannot know them all. So, when you go to the grocery store, always check nutritional fact labels to confirm if the food is low in sodium. Check for "sodium" on the food label and make sure the foods sodium content is equal to or less than 8% of your daily value. Foods containing more than 8% of your daily value of sodium per serving may not be good for your kidney health.

3. Go for fresh foods and homemade foods

Eating fresh foods reduces your sodium intake as fresh foods contain low sodium. In addition, go for homemade foods instead of packaged foods that may contain added sodium. When the food is homemade, you will be able to control the sodium content to suit your dietary needs. Eat fresh meat, beef, veal, pork, poultry, fish, vegetables, fruits, homemade soup, homemade broth, homemade sauce and so on.

4. **Always pay attention to serving size**

Most foods have a common serving size and their nutritional fact is usually estimated base on their specified serving size. Thus, it is not advisable for a chronic kidney disease patient to consume more than the given serving size of a food as this may cause excessive consumption of sodium even when the food has low sodium. For instance, if the serving size of a food is 100 grams and the sodium content per serving is 7% of your daily value, consuming 200 gram of that particular food per serving means you have consumed 14% of your daily value of sodium in one serving. Consuming 14% of your daily value of sodium intake at one serving is bad for your kidney health. There are common serving sizes; however, it is advisable that you go and consult a kidney dietitian to know the right serving size you are allowed to consume per meal for each food category according to the conditions of your kidneys.

5. **Consume low sodium foods moderately**

This is related to the issue of serving size. The fact that a food contains low sodium does not mean you should consume it excessively.

6. **Use herb and spices to cook instead of salt or salt seasonings**

Cultivate the habit of cooking without adding additional salt or salt seasonings. Rather, season your foods with herbs and spices moderately.

7. Go for unsalted foods

Check for phrases and words such as "no salt added" "unsalted" "sodium free" or "no sodium" on food packages. Food labeled with such words or phrases are usually safe to eat.

Potassium

Potassium is another essential electrolyte that performs important functions in our body. Potassium performs essential functions like supporting heart health, improving nerves and muscle functions, supporting bone health, balancing the fluid in and around our cells. When your kidneys are no longer functioning properly, they will be unable to get rid of excess potassium in the blood. This will result in an unhealthy buildup of potassium in your blood. An abnormal increase in blood potassium level is medically referred to as hyperkaliemia. Reducing your potassium consumption as a chronic disease is very important as hyperkaliemia can cause a lot of damages to your body. Consuming excess potassium can stress your unhealthy kidneys and make them worn out faster. In addition, excess build up of potassium in your blood stream as a result of the ineffectiveness of your kidneys can lead to low blood pressure- a negative health condition that can cause more damages to your kidneys. Generally, chronic kidney disease patients should not consume more than 1500 to 2300 milligrams of potassium per day. However, you may need to visit a kidney dietician to be sure of the right amount of potassium you should consume per day, depending on your kidney conditions and other variables.

How to regulate your potassium intake:

1. **Stay away from salt substitutes and seasonings that contain potassium**

Most salt substitutes and some seasonings contain potassium. Seasoning your food with salt substitutes or seasonings while cooking can result in excess potassium intake. Moreover, you should stay away from packages foods that contain salt substitute and potassium seasonings.

2. **Limit the consumption of high potassium foods**

All the foods we eat contain potassium; however, the potassium level of foods varies. Some foods are considered low in potassium while some are considered high in potassium. Foods that contain more than 200 mg of potassium per serving are considered high in potassium. As a chronic kidney disease patient, you have to limit your intake of high potassium foods and eat more low potassium foods. The list of high potassium foods include:

Fruits

Avocado, banana, medjool date, dried fruits, orange and orange juice, raisins, apricot, prunes and prune juice, pomegranate and pomegranate juice, sultanas, pumpkin, papaya, mango, nectarines, kiwi, honeydew melon, cantaloupe, fresh peaches, fresh pears, figs and melons.

Vegetables

Tomato, mushrooms, spinach, beetroot, dried beans, black kidney beans, pinto red beans, white beans, refried beans, chard, mustard, kale, spinach, turnip, collard, mustard, parsnips, yams, zucchini, winter squash, potatoes, artichokes, rutabagas, fried onions, broccoli, Brussels sprouts, kohlrabi, lentil and vegetable juice.

Nuts

Nuts are generally high in sodium.

Others

Processed meats, chocolate, puddings, yogurts, salt substitutes, peanut butter, nut butters, milk drinks, milk shakes, lentils, milk (evaporated milk, malted milk, soy milk, buttermilk), miso, seeds, tofu, creamed soups, ice cream, French fries, coconut, bran products, molasses, split peas , potato waffles, Hash browns and potato chips.

3. Eat more of low potassium foods

Your daily meals should feature more of low potassium foods. Such low potassium foods include:

Fruits

Apples, strawberry and strawberry nectar, pineapple, pineapple juice, apple sauce, apple juice, lime, raspberries, cranberry, cranberry juice, grape, grape juice, blueberries, blackberries, watermelon, tangerine, plums, mandarin oranges and fruit cocktail.

Vegetables

Carrots, onion, peas (green), alfalfa sprouts, eggplant, green beans, wax beans, lettuce, raw white mushrooms, peppers, cauliflower, cabbage, asparagus, celery, corn, radish, watercress, water chestnuts, cucumber, yellow squash, summer squash, okra, parsley, lemon and crookneck squash.

Other

Tortillas, rice, pasta, noodles, breads (excluding whole grain bread), alfafa seeds, regular oatmeal

4. **Eat fresh and homemade food**

Cooking at home and eating fresh foods gives you the opportunity to control your potassium intake. Packaged and processed foods may contain excess potassium.

5. **Check food nutritional labels**

Check nutritional labels on food packages to know their potassium content. Go for foods that contain less than 200 milligrams of potassium per serving. Foods containing more than 200 milligrams of potassium per serving may not be good for your kidney health.

6. **Pay attention to serving size**

Portion control is very important when following a renal diet. Do not consume more than one serving size of a food in one meal to avoid excess potassium intake. It is also advisable to visit a kidney dietician to know your perfect serving size for each food category, depending on your kidney condition and your body potassium level.

Phosphorous

Phosphorous is found in all foods and it is essential for our bones and muscle health. The kidneys are saddled with the responsibility of getting rid of excess phosphorous in our blood. Thus, when your kidneys are not healthy, excess phosphorous will start building up in your blood. Excess phosphorus will start extracting calcium from your bones, thereby causing severe bone weakness. To avoid this, you need to limit your phosphorous consumption if you have chronic kidney disease (CKD). Generally, chronic kidney disease patients should limit their phosphorous to 800 to 1000 milligrams per day. You should visit a kidney dietician to be sure of the right amount of potassium you are allowed to consume daily depending on the condition of your kidneys and other variables.

How to regulate your phosphorus consumption

1. **Limit the consumption of foods that contain high phosphorous**

All the foods we eat contain phosphorous; however, the amount of phosphorous content in food varies. Some foods contain high phosphorous content and some feature medium to low phosphorous. Foods containing less than 150 milligrams of phosphorous per serving have low phosphorous content, those containing 151 milligrams to 200 milligrams per serving are categorized under medium phosphorous foods and foods containing more than 200 milligrams per serving are considered to be high phosphorous foods. Chronic kidney disease patients should limit their consumption of high phosphorous foods. The list of high phosphorous foods includes:

Dairy and milk products

Goat cheese, part skim ricotta cheese, Romano cheese, parmesan cheese, buttermilk, chocolate milk, 1% milk, whole milk, low fat yogurt, skin yogurt, pudding, eggnog, soy milk, cream soup, custard, milk casseroles, condensed milk, evaporate milk, milk shake, non dairy creamers, processed cheese and non fat milk

Meat and protein foods

Pork, beef, tofu, beef liver, chicken liver, veal, lamb, organ meat, fish roe, processed meats, soy beans, beans, lentils, chickpeas, quinoa, amaranth and beefalo

Seafood

Fried calamari, oyster, sardine, blue mussels, crab clams, canned salmon, sole, swordfish, white tuna, light tuna, halibut, flounder, scallops and clam chowder

Beverages

Colas, beer, bottled ice tea, bottled fruit, punch and ale

Nuts and seeds

Almonds, peanuts, pine nuts, Brazil nuts, pecans, walnuts, pistachios, sunflower seeds, pumpkin seeds, chia seeds and cashews.

Others

Bran cereal, corn bread, wheat bread, whole grain breads, wheat flour and whole grain flour

2. **Check ingredient labels on package foods**

Take your time to check out for phosphorous or for words containing the morpheme "phos' on ingredient labels. Once you see phosphorous or any word containing "phos" on a food's ingredient labels, it means that the food contains added phosphorous. Please do your kidneys a favor by avoiding such packaged foods.

3. Consume high protein foods moderately

Protein rich foods naturally contain phosphorous. Foods that are high in protein usually contain high phosphorous content. Thus, high protein foods such as meat, dairy products, fish, poultry, nuts and beans should be consumed in smaller portions.

4. Use phosphate binders

Phosphate binders help to regulate the absorption of phosphorous in the foods we eat during digestion. Thus, taking phosphate binders at meal time can be used to control phosphorous consumption in CKD patients. However, you should consult a doctor or kidney dietician before using phosphate binders.

5. Check food nutritional fact labels

Check the nutritional fact labels on packaged foods. Select foods that contain less than 10% of your daily value of phosphorous intake. This may not be relevant in all cases as most food nutritional fact labels do not include phosphorous, even though the food contains phosphorous.

6. Pay attention to serving size

Do not consume more than one serving size of a food in a single meal. Eating more than one serving size of a low phosphorous food at a single meal can make a low phosphorous food become a high phosphorous food. Most foods have a common serving size; however, you may need to consult a dietician to know your perfect serving size for each food group.

7. Eat homemade and fresh foods

Cooking at home and eating fresh foods keeps you in control of your phosphorous consumption. You will be able to choose which foods to include in your meal, avoid phosphorous addictives and pay attention to serving size. Eating too much of packaged foods may not be good for kidneys.

Protein

Chronic kidney patients (CKD) also need to regulate their protein consumption. Protein is an essential macronutrient; it is need by our body to build muscles, fight infections, build tissues and heal wounds. People with healthy kidneys can eat high protein meals because their kidneys are active enough to excrete protein waste. However, CKD patients are advised to limit their protein intake as high protein intake can increase waste products in the blood and stress the kidneys. Limiting protein intake can be a bit tricky as insufficient intake of protein can also trigger some negative health conditions. Our body protein needs is determined by factors such as body size, sex and age. To stay safe, you need to consult a doctor or a kidney dietician to know the right amount of protein you should consume per day.

Fluid

Chronic kidney disease patient will also need to limit their daily consumption of liquids/fluids. Unhealthy kidneys do not have the capacity to effectively excrete excess body fluids. Thus, excess fluid will start to build up in the blood. The buildup of excess fluid in the blood can cause high blood pressure – a negative health condition that can accelerate the loss of kidney functions. This can also result in edema (swollen arms, joint, ankles, feet and legs).

CHAPTER FOUR

Kidney friendly Homemade Kitchen Staples and Seasonings

Beef Stock

PREP TIME: 5 minutes

COOK TIME: 4 hours 30 minutes

SERVINGS: 8 cups

Ingredients:

- 2 tbsp olive oil
- 9 cups water
- 2 pound beef bones (all fat trimmed)
- 2 fresh parsley stems
- ½ tsp curry powder
- ½ tsp thyme
- 2 celery stalks (chopped)
- 2 carrots (boiled without salt, drained and chopped)
- 1 tsp black peppercorns
- 1 bay leaf

Directions:

1. Preheat the oven to 440°F.
2. Arrange the beef bones into a deep baking pan and place the baking pan in the preheated oven.
3. Bake the beef bones for about 30 minutes.

4. Remove the baking pan from the oven. Add 1 tbsp olive oil and toss.
5. Add the carrot and celery.
6. Return the baking pan to the oven and bake the beef bones for another 30 minutes.
7. After the baking cycle, remove the baking pan from the oven and pour the roasted beef bones and veggies into saucepan.
8. Pour in the water and stir the parsley, black peppercorn, curry and thyme.
9. Add bay leave and bring the liquid to a boil over medium to high heat. Reduce the heat low and simmer the broth for 3 hours, covered. Check the broth at interval to skim off any foam or dirt that rises to the surface of the broth.
10. Remove the sauce pan from heat and leave the broth to cool for about 25 minutes.
11. Discard the bay leaf and strain the broth into a clean bowl with a fine mesh strainer.
12. Pour broth into containers and store in a refrigerator for up to six days. Always skim off excess fat from the surface of the broth before using.

Nutrition Facts
Servings: 8

Amount per serving
Calories 195

% Daily Value*

Total Fat 8.9g	**11%**
Saturated Fat 2.5g	**13%**
Cholesterol 76mg	**25%**
Sodium 76mg	**3%**
Total Carbohydrate 1.6g	**1%**
Dietary Fiber 0.7g	**2%**
Total Sugars 0.5g	
Protein 26.1g	
Vitamin D 0mcg	0%
Calcium 21mg	2%
Iron 16mg	91%
Potassium 60mg	

Relish

PREP TIME: 20 minutes

SERVINGS: 36 (1 tbsp per serving)

Ingredients:

- 1 cup chopped cucumber
- ¼ tsp cinnamon
- 1/8 tsp cayenne pepper
- 1 tsp celery seed
- 1/8 tsp allspice
- 1 large onion (chopped)
- 2 cups chopped celery
- ½ cup sugar
- ¼ tsp ground mustard
- 1 small green pepper (chopped)
- 4 tbsp fresh chopped cilantro

Directions:

1. In a large mixing bowl, combine the cucumber, green pepper, cilantro, onion and celery.
2. Add the sugar, cinnamon, allspice, cayenne and mustard. Toss until the ingredients are well combined.
3. Cover the mixing bowl and place it in a mixing bowl. Chill for about 8 hours.

Nutrition Facts
Serving size: 1 tablespoon
Servings: 36

Amount per serving
Calories 14

% Daily Value*

Total Fat 0g	0%
Saturated Fat 0g	0%
Cholesterol 0mg	0%
Sodium 5mg	0%
Total Carbohydrate 3.6g	1%
Dietary Fiber 0.3g	1%
Total Sugars 3.1g	
Protein 0.1g	
Vitamin D 0mcg	0%
Calcium 5mg	0%
Iron 0mg	0%
Potassium 30mg	

Vegetable Stock

PREP TIME: 5 minutes

COOK TIME: 2 hours

SERVINGS: 6 cups

Ingredients:

- 7 cups of water
- 1 tsp black peppercorns
- 2 carrots (peeled and sliced)
- 1 onion (chopped)
- 4 garlic cloves (cloves)
- 4 celery stalks (chopped)
- 2 bay leaves
- 3 sprigs thyme
- 3 parsley sprigs

Directions:

1. Combine the water, parsley, garlic, onion, celery, bay leaves, peppercorns, carrots and thyme in a large sauce pan over medium to high heat.
2. Bring the mixture to a boil; cover the sauce pan; reduce the heat to medium-low and simmer the broth for about 2 hours, checking occasionally to skim off any fat that rises to the surface of the broth.
3. Remove the sauce pan from heat and discard the bay leaves.
4. Strain the vegetable broth into a clean bowl with a fine mesh strainer.

5. Pour the broth into jars and let it cool completely before sealing the jars.
6. Store the vegetable stock in the refrigerator for up to 5 days.

Nutrition Facts

Servings: 6

Amount per serving

Calories 24

% Daily Value*

Total Fat 0.1g 0%

  Saturated Fat 0g 0%

Cholesterol 0mg 0%

Sodium 33mg 1%

Total Carbohydrate 5.4g 2%

  Dietary Fiber 1.5g 5%

  Total Sugars 2g

Protein 0.7g

Vitamin D 0mcg 0%

Calcium 41mg 3%

Iron 1mg 6%

Potassium 144mg

Chicken Stock

PREP TIME: 5 minutes

COOK TIME: 2 hours

SERVINGS: 6 cups

Ingredients:

- 7 cups of water
- 2 pounds whole chicken (raw) cut into small bite sizes
- 1 bay leaf
- 1 black peppercorns
- 1 carrot (sliced)
- 1 onion (chopped)
- 4 celery stalks (chopped)
- 5 fresh thyme sprigs
- 3 fresh parsley stems

Directions:

1. Combine the chicken meat, thyme, celery, parsley, peppercorns, onion, carrot, bay leaf and water in a large sauce pan over medium to high heat.
2. Bring the mixture to a boil; reduce the heat to low and simmer the stock for about 2 hour, covered. Check the stock occasionally to skim off any foam or dirt on the surface of the stock.
3. Remove the sauce pan from heat and discard the bay leaf.
4. Strain the chicken stock into a clean bowl with a fine mesh strainer.

5. Pour the chicken stock into jars and let it cool completely before sealing the jars.
6. Store the chicken stock in a refrigerator for up to 7 days.

Nutrition Facts	
Servings: 6	
Amount per serving	
Calories	**190**
	% Daily Value*
Total Fat 11.5g	15%
Saturated Fat 3.4g	17%
Cholesterol 67mg	22%
Sodium 81mg	4%
Total Carbohydrate 3.5g	1%
Dietary Fiber 1.1g	4%
Total Sugars 1.5g	
Protein 14.6g	
Vitamin D 0mcg	0%
Calcium 42mg	3%
Iron 1mg	8%
Potassium 121mg	

Barbeque Sauce

PREP TIME: 5 minutes

COOK TIME: 5minutes

SERVINGS: 8 (2 tbsp per serving)

Ingredients:

- 5 tbsp + 1 tsp canola oil
- ¼ tsp onion powder
- 1 tbsp brown sugar
- ¼ cup vinegar
- 1 tbsp paprika
- ½ cup unsalted tomato juice
- 1 clove garlic (crushed)
- 1/3 cup water
- 1 tsp pepper

Directions:

1. Combine all the ingredients in a sauce pan.
2. Bring the mixture to a boil, reduce the heat and simmer the sauce for 20 minutes.
3. Pour leftover into a tightly sealed container and store in a refrigerator.

Nutrition Facts
Servings: 8

Amount per serving
Calories 95

% Daily Value*

Total Fat 9.4g	**12%**
Saturated Fat 0.7g	**4%**
Cholesterol 0mg	**0%**
Sodium 3mg	**0%**
Total Carbohydrate 2.7g	**1%**
Dietary Fiber 0.5g	**2%**
Total Sugars 1.8g	
Protein 0.3g	
Vitamin D 0mcg	0%
Calcium 7mg	1%
Iron 0mg	2%
Potassium 68mg	

Alfredo Sauce

PREP TIME: 10 minutes

COOK TIME: 10 minutes

SERVINGS: 8 (¼ cup per serving)

Ingredients:

- 2 tbsp butter (unsalted)
- ¼ tsp ground nutmeg
- 1 cup plain rice milk (rice milk)
- 1 ½ tbsp all purpose flour
- ¾ cup plain cream cheese
- 1 garlic clove (minced)
- 2 tbsp parmesan cheese
- ½ tsp ground black pepper

Directions:

1. Melt the butter in a sauce pan over medium heat.
2. Stir in the flour and minced garlic. Cook for about 2 minutes, stirring constantly.
3. Stir in the rice milk. Cook for about 4 minutes or until is thick, stirring constantly.
4. Add the cream cheese, nutmeg and parmesan cheese. Stir to combine and cook for 1 minute, stirring constantly until the sauce is smooth.
5. Remove the sauce pan from heat and stir in the ground black pepper.
6. Serve hot over kidney friendly pasta.

Nutrition Facts
Servings: 8

Amount per serving
Calories 123

% Daily Value*

Total Fat 9.8g	13%
Saturated Fat 6g	30%
Cholesterol 29mg	10%
Sodium 109mg	5%
Total Carbohydrate 7.6g	3%
Dietary Fiber 0.1g	0%
Total Sugars 2.9g	
Protein 3.1g	
Vitamin D 0mcg	1%
Calcium 100mg	8%
Iron 0mg	1%
Potassium 5mg	

Cinnamon Apple Sauce

PREP TIME: 10 minutes

COOK TIME: 30 minutes

SERVINGS: 6 servings (½ per serving)

Ingredients:

- 8 apples (peeled, cored and cut into chunks)
- 1/8 tsp ground all spice
- ½ cup water
- 1 tsp ground cinnamon
- ¼ tsp ground nutmeg
- ¼ tsp ground ginger

Directions:

1. Combine the apples, water, nutmeg, ginger, cinnamon and allspice in a large sauce pan over medium heat.
2. Cover the sauce pan and cook for about 15 to 20 minutes or until the apples are tender, stirring occasionally.
3. Remove the sauce from heat and use a potato mash to mash the apples.
4. Let the sauce cool completely before transferring it to jars for storage. Store in a refrigerator for up to 7 days.

Nutrition Facts
Servings: 6

Amount per serving
Calories 12

% Daily Value*

Total Fat 0.1g	0%
Saturated Fat 0g	0%
Cholesterol 0mg	0%
Sodium 1mg	0%
Total Carbohydrate 3.2g	1%
Dietary Fiber 0.5g	**2%**
Total Sugars 2.2g	
Protein 0.1g	
Vitamin D 0mcg	0%
Calcium 6mg	0%
Iron 0mg	0%
Potassium 23mg	

Italian Seasoning

PREP TIME: 5 minutes

SERVINGS: 24 (1/2 cup – 1 tsp per serving)

Ingredients:

- 2 tsp onion powder
- 1 tbsp oregano
- 2 tbsp garlic powder
- 1 tbsp parsley
- 1 tbsp basil
- 1/2tsp pepper
- ½ tsp thyme

Directions:

1. Combine all the ingredients in a small mixing bowl. Stir thoroughly until the ingredients are well combined.
2. Store in an airtight container.

Nutrition Facts
Servings: 24

Amount per serving
Calories 4

% Daily Value*

Total Fat 0g	**0%**
Saturated Fat 0g	**0%**
Cholesterol 0mg	**0%**
Sodium 0mg	**0%**
Total Carbohydrate 0.8g	**0%**
Dietary Fiber 0.2g	**1%**
Total Sugars 0.3g	
Protein 0.2g	
Vitamin D 0mcg	0%
Calcium 5mg	0%
Iron 0mg	1%
Potassium 15mg	

Breakfast

Blueberry Pancake

PREP TIME: 10 minutes

COOK TIME: 24 minutes

SERVINGS: 12 pancakes

Ingredients:

- 2 tbsp canola oil
- 2 eggs (beaten)
- 1 1/2cups sifted plain all purpose flour
- 1 cup buttermilk
- 1 tsp ground cinnamon
- 1 cup frozen blueberries (rinsed)
- 2 tsp Ener-G baking powder (or any other renal friendly sodium free baking powder)
- 3 tbsp sugar

Directions:

1. Sift the cinnamon, all-purpose flour and sugar into a large mixing bowl. Mix until the ingredients are well combined.
2. Use a spoon to make a hole in the middle of the mixture. Pour in the egg and buttermilk and mix until the mixture forms a smooth batter.
3. Fold in the rinsed blueberries.
4. Heat up a large pan and add little oil. Pour ½ cup of the batter into the pan.
5. Cook for about 1 to 2 minutes. Flip the pancake and cook the other side for about 1 to 2 minute too.

6. Repeat step 4 and 5 until all the batter has been cooked.
7. Serve and enjoy.

Nutrition Facts
Servings: 12

Amount per serving
Calories 164

% Daily Value*

Total Fat 3.4g	4%
Saturated Fat 0.5g	3%
Cholesterol 28mg	9%
Sodium 35mg	2%
Total Carbohydrate 30.2g	11%
Dietary Fiber 0.8g	3%
Total Sugars 5.3g	
Protein 2.1g	
Vitamin D 3mcg	13%
Calcium 204mg	16%
Iron 0mg	3%
Potassium 51mg	

Vegetable Omelet

PREP TIME: 5 minutes

COOK TIME: 5 minutes

SERVINGS: 1

Ingredients:

- 1 tbsp canola oil
- 1 whole egg
- 2 egg whites
- 2 tbsp water
- 1/3 cup frozen mixed vegetables
- 4 tbsp sliced green pepper
- ½ cup diced onion
  Garnish:
- 2 fresh parsley sprigs (chopped)

Directions:

1. Cut the mixed vegetables into pieces and put them in a microwave safe dish. Add little water and cover the dish.
2. Place the dish in the microwave and microwave on HIGH for 2 minutes.
3. Remove the dish from the vegetables from the microwave and set them aside in a bowl.
4. Heat up the oil in a small nonstick skillet.
5. Add the onion and green pepper. Saute for about 2 minutes, stirring often.
6. Beat the egg, egg whites and water in a mixing bowl.
7. Pour the egg mixture into the skillet and cook until the egg is set and firm.

8. Add the mixed steamed mix vegetables and fold the omelet.
9. Remove the pan from heat.
10. Serve the omelet into plate and garnish with chop parsley.

Nutrition Facts

Servings: 1

Amount per serving

Calories	270
	% Daily Value*
Total Fat 18.7g	24%
Saturated Fat 2.4g	12%
Cholesterol 164mg	55%
Sodium 216mg	9%
Total Carbohydrate 12g	4%
Dietary Fiber 3.3g	12%
Total Sugars 5.1g	
Protein 14.6g	
Vitamin D 15mcg	77%
Calcium 56mg	4%
Iron 1mg	8%
Potassium 378mg	

Pumpkin Pancake

PREP TIME: 10 minutes

COOK TIME: 15 minutes

SERVINGS: 8

Ingredients:

- 3 tbsp canola oil
- 2 cups gluten free baking flour
- 1 large egg (beaten)
- 1 tsp pure vanilla extract
- 2 tbsp pure maple syrup
- 1 tbsp Ener-G baking powder
- ½ tsp Ener-G baking soda
- 2 tbsp ground flax seeds
- ½ cup pumpkin puree (unsweetened)
- 1 ½ cup unsweetened almond milk
- ¼ tsp salt
- 1 tsp cinnamon

Directions:

1. In a large mixing bowl, combine the flour, baking powder, flax seeds, baking powder, cinnamon, salt and baking soda.
2. In another large mixing bowl, whisk together the egg, milk, vanilla extract, pumpkin puree and maple syrup.
3. Gently pour the wet ingredients into the dry ingredient, mixing as you pour in the wet ingredient. Mix until well combined and smooth.
4. Heat up a large skillet over medium to high heat.

5. Lightly oil the pan.
6. Pour about 1/3 cup of the batter into the pan.
7. Cook for about 1 to 2 minutes and flip. Cook the other side for about 1 to 2 minutes too.
8. Transfer the pancake to a neat plate.
9. Repeat the cooking process until all the batter has been cooked into pancakes.
10. Serve warm and enjoy.

Nutrition Facts

Servings: 8

Amount per serving

Calories 173

% Daily Value*

Total Fat 7.1g	9%
Saturated Fat 0.7g	4%
Cholesterol 23mg	8%
Sodium 118mg	5%
Total Carbohydrate 24.2g	9%
Dietary Fiber 2g	7%
Total Sugars 3.7g	
Protein 2.3g	
Vitamin D 2mcg	12%
Calcium 525mg	40%
Iron 4mg	22%
Potassium 102mg	

Granola Breakfast Bowl

PREP TIME: 10 minutes

COOK TIME: 25 minutes

SERVINGS: 5

Ingredients:

- 2 cups rolled oat
- ½ cup natural honey
- ¼ cup bee pollen
- 1 tsp vanilla extract
- ½ tsp salt or to taste
- 1 cup unsweetened reduced coconut flakes
- 3 tbsp coconut sugar
- 1 tsp cinnamon
- ¼ cup melted coconut oil
- ½ cup pecans (roughly chopped)
- ½ cup almonds (roughly chopped)
  Topping:
- Almond milk

Directions:

1. Preheat your oven to 175°C.
2. Line a baking sheet with parchment paper, set aside.
3. Toss the oat into a large mixing bowl and add the chopped pecans, chopped almond, coconut sugar, coconut flakes, salt and cinnamon. Mix until the ingredients are evenly combined.
4. In another mixing bowl, mix the melted coconut oil, honey and vanilla extract.

5. Now, pour the honey mixture into the oat mixture and stir thoroughly until the ingredients are well combined.
6. Place the mixture on the line baking sheet and spread evenly, leveling the surface of the granola.
7. Place the baking sheet in the oven and bake for 15 minutes.
8. Remove the baking sheet from the oven and toss the granola mixture.
9. Return the baking sheet to the oven and bake for another 10 minutes.
10. Sprinkle the bee pollen over the roasted granola mixture and mix.
11. Lay parchment paper over the roasted granola and gently press the granola to the bottom of the baking sheet.
12. Remove and discard the parchment paper.
13. Leave the granola to cool for a few minutes.
14. Serve into bowls, top with almond milk and enjoy.

Nutrition Facts
Servings: 5

Amount per serving
Calories 518

% Daily Value*

Total Fat 34.5g	**44%**
Saturated Fat 9.1g	**45%**
Cholesterol 0mg	**0%**
Sodium 327mg	**14%**
Total Carbohydrate 44.1g	**16%**
Dietary Fiber 8.7g	**31%**
Total Sugars 3.2g	
Protein 10.1g	
Vitamin D 0mcg	0%
Calcium 63mg	5%
Iron 2mg	13%
Potassium 282mg	

Simple Cumin Raisin Breakfast Quinoa

PREP TIME: 5 minutes

COOK TIME: 17 minutes

SERVINGS: 8

Ingredients:

- 2 cups quinoa
- ½ cup raisins
- 2 tbsp cumin
- 4 cups vegetable broth
- 1 tbsp olive oil
- 1/2 tsp ground black pepper
- 1 small yellow onion (diced)

Garnish:

- 2 tbsp freshly chopped cilantro

Directions:

1. Heat up a pot on high heat and add oil.
2. Add the onions and saute until tender and lightly browned. This will take about 2 minutes.
3. Stir in the cumin, salt and pepper.
4. Pour in the broth and add the quinoa and raisin. Bring to a boil; reduce the heat and simmer for 10 to 15 minutes more.
5. Serve into bowls and garnish with chopped fresh cilantro.

Nutrition Facts
Servings: 8

Amount per serving
Calories 227

% Daily Value*

Total Fat 5.4g | **7%**
Saturated Fat 0.8g | **4%**
Cholesterol 0mg | **0%**
Sodium 388mg | **17%**
Total Carbohydrate 36.5g | **13%**
Dietary Fiber 3.7g | **13%**
Total Sugars 6.1g
Protein 9.1g

Vitamin D 0mcg | 0%
Calcium 46mg | 4%
Iron 3mg | 19%
Potassium 453mg

Blueberry Breakfast Smoothie Bowl

PREP TIME: 5 minutes

SERVINGS: 1 bowl

Ingredients:

- 1 cup frozen blueberries
- ½ tsp ginger
- ½ medium apple (peeled and slices)
- 1 tbsp fiber cereal
- 2 tbsp whey protein powder
- 100 g fat free Greek yogurt
- 1/3 cup unsweetened almond milk
- 5 raspberries
- 2 strawberries (sliced)
- 2 tsp shredded coconut

Directions:

1. Put blueberries and apple in a blender and blend until just smooth.
2. Add the almond milk, fiber cereal, protein powder, ginger and Greek yoghurt. Blend until smooth.
3. Serve the smoothie into bowl and top with shredded coconut, raspberry and strawberry

Nutrition Facts
Servings: 1

Amount per serving
Calories 347

% Daily Value*

Total Fat 5.6g	**7%**
Saturated Fat 1.9g	**10%**
Cholesterol 57mg	**19%**
Sodium 171mg	**7%**
Total Carbohydrate 54g	**20%**
Dietary Fiber 12.6g	**45%**
Total Sugars 27.8g	
Protein 26.3g	
Vitamin D 0mcg	2%
Calcium 140mg	11%
Iron 5mg	27%
Potassium 583mg	

Blueberry Muffin

PREP TIME: 15 minutes

COOK TIME: 30 minutes

SERVINGS: 12 muffins

Ingredients:

- 1/8 tsp ground ginger
- ½ cup canola oil
- 1 cup granulated sugar
- 2 cups fresh blueberries
- 2 cups unsweetened rice milk
- 2 tbsp pure vanilla extract
- 1 tbsp Ener-G baking soda (or any other renal friendly sodium free baking powder)
- ½ tsp ground nutmeg
- 1 tsp cinnamon
- 3 ½ cups all-purpose flour

Directions:

1. Preheat the oven to 375°F and line 12 muffin cups with parchment paper.
2. In a large mixing bowl, combine the all-purpose flour, nutmeg, cinnamon, baking powder, ginger and sugar. Mix until the ingredients are well combined.
3. In another large mixing bowl, combine the vanilla extract, rice milk and canola oil. Mix until well combined.
4. Now, pour the milk mixture into the flour mixture and mix until you form a smooth batter.
5. Fold in the blueberries.

6. Fill each muffin cup with the batter. The muffin cups should not be filled to the beam; leave at least 1 inch empty.
7. Arrange the muffin cups into a baking sheet and place the baking sheet into the oven.
8. Bake for about 25 minutes to 30 minutes or until a toothpick inserted in the middle of the muffin comes out clean.
9. Remove the muffins from the oven and leave them to cool.
10. Remove the muffins from the muffin cups and serve.
11. Enjoy.

Nutrition Facts
Servings: 12

Amount per serving

Calories 317

% Daily Value*

Total Fat 10g	**13%**
Saturated Fat 0.8g	**4%**
Cholesterol 0mg	**0%**
Sodium 18mg	**1%**
Total Carbohydrate 52.3g	**19%**
Dietary Fiber 1.7g	**6%**
Total Sugars 21.1g	
Protein 4.1g	
Vitamin D 0mcg	1%
Calcium 71mg	5%
Iron 2mg	12%
Potassium 66mg	

Overnight French toast

PREP TIME: 20 minutes

COOK TIME: 50 minutes

SERVINGS: 9

Ingredients:

- 1 loaf of white bread (cut into 1 inch slices)
- ½ cup unsweetened dried blueberries
- 1 tbsp vanilla
- 3 tsp cinnamon
- 1 tsp nutmeg
- 3 apples (peeled, cored, and finely chopped)
- 1 ½ cups unsweetened rice milk
- 6 eggs
- ½ cup margarine (unsalted)
- 1 cup brown sugar

Directions:

1. Whisk together the brown sugar, 1 tsp cinnamon, nutmeg and mayonnaise in a 13 by 9 inch dish.
2. Add the blueberries and apple. Toss until well combined.
3. Toss until the ingredients are well combined.
4. Spread the mixture and press it to the bottom of the baking dish.
5. Arrange with bread slices on the apple mixture.
6. In a large mixing bowl, whisk together the eggs, rice milk, 2 tsp cinnamon and vanilla.

7. Pour the egg mixture over the bread slices in the baking dish. Cover the baking dish with foil and place it in a refrigerator. Refrigerate the mixture overnight.
8. Preheat the oven to 375°F.
9. Place the baking dish in the oven and bake for about 40 minutes, covered.
10. Remove the baking dish from the oven and uncover the dish.
11. Return the dish to the oven and bake the toast for another 5 minutes.
12. After the baking cycle, remove the baking dish from the oven and let the toast cool for about 5 minutes.
13. Serve the French toast and enjoy.

Nutrition Facts
Servings: 9

Amount per serving
Calories 588

% Daily Value*

Total Fat 26.1g	**33%**
Saturated Fat 4.5g	**23%**
Cholesterol 109mg	**36%**
Sodium 500mg	**22%**
Total Carbohydrate 75.9g	**28%**
Dietary Fiber 3.6g	**13%**
Total Sugars 32.1g	
Protein 11.6g	
Vitamin D 10mcg	52%
Calcium 224mg	17%
Iron 4mg	20%
Potassium 174mg	

Cinnamon Bran Muffins

PREP TIME: 10 minutes

COOK TIME: 20 minutes

SERVINGS: 12

Ingredients:

- 1 tsp cinnamon
- 1 egg
- 1 tsp pure vanilla extract
- 1 ½ tsp Ener-G sodium free baking soda (or any other kidney friendly sodium free baking soda)
- 1/3 cup natural honey
- 1 cup wheat bran
- ¼ tsp cream of tartar
- 1 cup crushed pineapple (drained)
- 1cup all-purpose flour

Directions:

1. Preheat the oven to 400°F and grease 12 muffin cups.
2. In a large mixing bowl, combine the cinnamon, all-purpose flour, wheat bran, cream of tartar and baking soda.
3. In another large mixing, combine the crushed pineapple, honey, egg and vanilla extract.
4. Now, pour the flour mixture into the egg mixture and mix until you form a smooth barter.
5. Fill each muffin cup with the batter. The muffin cups should not be filled to the beam; leave at least 1 inch empty.

6. Arrange the muffin cups into a baking sheet and place the baking sheet into the oven.
7. Bake for about 25 minutes to 30 minutes or until a toothpick inserted in the middle of the muffin comes out clean.
8. Remove the muffins from the oven and leave them to cool.
9. Remove the muffins from the muffin cups and serve.
10. Enjoy.

Nutrition Facts
Servings: 12

Amount per serving
Calories 63

% Daily Value*

Total Fat 0.6g	1%
Saturated Fat 0.1g	1%
Cholesterol 14mg	5%
Sodium 5mg	0%
Total Carbohydrate 13.3g	5%
Dietary Fiber 2.7g	10%
Total Sugars 2.2g	
Protein 2.3g	
Vitamin D 1mcg	6%
Calcium 16mg	1%
Iron 1mg	6%
Potassium 88mg	

Corn Pudding

PREP TIME: 10 minutes

COOK TIME: 40 minutes

SERVINGS: 6

Ingredients:

- 2 tbsp granulated sugar
- 3 eggs (beaten)
- 2 tbsp all-purpose flour
- ½ tsp Ener-G baking soda (or any other renal friendly sodium free baking soda)
- ¾ cup rice milk (unsweetened)
- 2 cups frozen corn kernels (defrosted)
- 2 tbsp sour cream
- 1 tsp pure vanilla extract
- 3 tbsp unsalted butter (softened)
- 1 tsp ginger powder

Directions:

1. Preheat your oven to 350°F and grease and 8 by 8 inch baking dish with butter.
2. In a large mixing bowl, combine the egg, rice milk, sugar, butter, sour cream and vanilla extract. Mix until the ingredients are well combined.
3. In another mixing bowl, combine the all-purpose flour, ginger baking soda.
4. Pour the flour mixture into the egg mixture and mix until you form a smooth batter.
5. Add the defrosted corn and mix until well combined.

6. Fill the prepared baking dish with the batter.
7. Place the baking dish in the preheated oven and bake for about 40 minutes.
8. After the baking cycle, remove the baking dish from the oven and let the pudding cool for about 12 to 15 minutes.
9. Serve the corn pudding into bowls and enjoy.

Nutrition Facts
Servings: 6

Amount per serving
Calories 177

% Daily Value*

Total Fat 9.5g	**12%**
Saturated Fat 4.9g	**25%**
Cholesterol 99mg	**33%**
Sodium 87mg	**4%**
Total Carbohydrate 19.9g	**7%**
Dietary Fiber 1.4g	**5%**
Total Sugars 7.3g	
Protein 4.8g	
Vitamin D 12mcg	59%
Calcium 62mg	5%
Iron 1mg	5%
Potassium 175mg	

Breakfast Meatballs

PREP TIME: 20 minutes

COOK TIME: 25 minutes

SERVINGS: 35 meatballs

Ingredients:

- 1pound lean ground turkey
- ¼ cup finely chopped onions
- 1tsp hot sauce
- ½ tsp garlic powder
- 1tsp sodium free poultry seasoning
- ¼ tsp dry mustard
- 1 tsp granulated sugar
- 1/2 tsp onion powder
- 1 tbsp fresh lemon juice
- 1 tsp Italian seasoning
  Sauce ingredients:
- 2 cups of water
- ¼ cup vegetable oil
- 1tsp curry
- 1 tsp hot sauce
- 2 tbsp all-purpose flour
- 2 tsp vinegar
- 1 tsp onion powder
  Garnish:
- Chopped fresh parsley (optional)

Directions:

1. Preheat your oven to 425°F and line a baking sheet with parchment paper.
2. In a large mixing bowl, combine the ground turkey, chopped onions, sugar lemon juice.
3. Add the Italian seasoning, onion powder, hot sauce, mustard, garlic powder and poultry seasoning. Mix until well combined.
4. Use a tablespoon to scoop out equal amount of the mixture and mold into balls.
5. Arrange the meatballs into the lined baking sheet in a single layer.
6. Place the baking sheet in the preheated oven and bake the meatballs for about 20 minutes or until the meatballs are done.
7. Meanwhile, prepare the sauce. Place a sauce pan on heat and add the vegetable oil and all-purpose flour.
8. Cook for a few minutes, stirring constantly until the mixture is slightly browned.
9. Remove the saucepan from heat and stir in the onion powder, hot sauce, water, curry and sugar.
10. Return the saucepan to heat and cook until the sauce thickens, stirring constantly. Remove the saucepan from heat.
11. After the baking cycle, remove the baking sheet from the oven and leave the meatballs to cool for a few minutes.
12. Serve the meatballs warm with the sauce and garnish with chopped fresh parsley.

Nutrition Facts
Servings: 35

Amount per serving
Calories 36

% Daily Value*

Total Fat 2.6g	**3%**
Saturated Fat 0.4g	**2%**
Cholesterol 9mg	**3%**
Sodium 18mg	**1%**
Total Carbohydrate 0.7g	**0%**
Dietary Fiber 0.1g	**0%**
Total Sugars 0.2g	
Protein 2.6g	
Vitamin D 0mcg	0%
Calcium 4mg	0%
Iron 0mg	1%
Potassium 48mg	1%

Breakfast Frittata

PREP TIME: 15 minutes

COOK TIME: 35 minutes

SERVINGS: 6

Ingredients:

- 8 eggs
- 1 tbsp vegetable oil
- 1 cup chopped asparagus
- 1/8 tsp garlic
- ¼ tsp onion powder
- 1/4 tsp salt
- ½ tsp ground black pepper
- 1/8 tsp cayenne pepper
- 1/8 tsp cumin
- 1/8 tsp coriander
- 1/8 tsp oregano
- 1 red bell pepper (seeded and chopped)
- ½ tsp dried basil
- ½ cup shredded Swiss cheese
- ½ cup rice milk
- 1 medium potato (peeled and cut into bite sizes) *See notes

Directions:

1. Put the potato pieces in a pot and add enough water.
2. Bring the water and potato to a boil.
3. Drain off the hot water and add fresh water.

4. Bring the fresh water and potatoes to a boil and cook until the potato pieces are tender.
5. Drain the water and set aside.
6. In a mixing bowl, whisk together the egg, basil, rice milk, oregano, coriander, cayenne pepper, black pepper, salt, onion powder and garlic. Set aside.
7. Heat up the vegetable oil in a frying pan over medium to high heat.
8. Add the chopped pepper and asparagus and saute until the vegetables are tender, stirring often.
9. Add the cooked potato pieces and stir. Spread out the veggies and potato across the pan.
10. Pour the egg mixture over the ingredients in the frying pan.
11. Cover the pan, reduce the heat and cook for about 15 minutes or until the eggs are set and the frittata is firm.
12. Sprinkle the Swiss cheese over the frittata after the first 13 minutes of cooking.
13. Remove the frying pan from heat and let the frittata cool for a few minutes.
14. Cut frittata into sizes and serve.

Note: it is important that you double cook the potatoes as instructed. Changing the water after the first boiling helps to reduce the potatoes' potassium content. Preparing this recipe without double boiling the potatoes will turn the meal into a high potassium meal.

Nutrition Facts
Servings: 6

Amount per serving
Calories 188

% Daily Value*

Total Fat 10.9g — **14%**

　Saturated Fat 3.9g — **20%**

Cholesterol 227mg — **76%**

Sodium 207mg — **9%**

Total Carbohydrate 11.9g — **4%**

　Dietary Fiber 1.6g — **6%**

　Total Sugars 2.3g

Protein 11.3g

Vitamin D 24mcg — 122%

Calcium 118mg — 9%

Iron 2mg — 11%

Potassium 329mg

Egg Sandwiches

PREP TIME: 5 minutes

COOK TIME: 20 minutes

SERVINGS: 6 sandwiches

Ingredients:

- 8 small eggs
- 12 slices of bread
- 2 green onions (chopped)
- ½ cup finely chopped celery
- 1/3 cup light sour cream
- 1 tbsp mayonnaise
- ¼ cup chopped green pepper
- 1/8 tsp paprika
- 1/8 tsp ground black pepper
- ¼ tsp ground mustard

Directions:

1. Place the eggs in a pot and add enough water.
2. Bring the egg and to a rolling boil over high heat, reduce the heat and cook for 15 minutes to ensure the eggs are hard boiled.
3. Remove eggs from heat and put them in a bowl of cold water for a few minutes. Peel the eggs.
4. Place the peeled eggs in a bowl and mash.
5. Now, add the mayonnaise, sour cream, paprika, green pepper, onion, celery and mustard. Mix until the ingredients are well combined.

6. Arrange six bread slices on a tray and spoon equal amount of the egg mixture onto the bread.
7. Spread the egg mixture and cover the bread slices with the remaining bread slices.
8. Serve and enjoy.

Nutrition Facts

Servings: 6

Amount per serving

Calories 162

% Daily Value*

Total Fat 9g	12%
Saturated Fat 3.5g	18%
Cholesterol 195mg	65%
Sodium 226mg	10%
Total Carbohydrate 11.5g	4%
Dietary Fiber 0.8g	3%
Total Sugars 1.9g	
Protein 8.4g	
Vitamin D 42mcg	208%
Calcium 79mg	6%
Iron 2mg	9%
Potassium 151mg	

Carrot Scramble

PREP TIME: 10 minutes

COOK TIME: 10 minutes

SERVINGS: 4

Ingredients:

- 2 tbsp olive oil
- 5 eggs (beaten)
- 1/4 tsp garlic powder
- 1/8 tsp basil
- 1/8 tsp pepper
- 1 cup chopped onion
- ½ cup nestle non dairy creamer
- 1 cup cooked carrot
- ½ medium red pepper (chopped)
- ¼ cup frozen corn (defrosted)

Directions:

1. Heat up the olive oil in a skillet over medium to high heat.
2. Add the onion and chopped pepper. Saute until the onion is browned and tender, stirring often.
3. Add the carrot, corn, pepper, garlic powder and basil. Stir and cook for about 2 minutes.
4. In a mixing bowl, whisk together the eggs and non dairy creamer.
5. Pour the egg mixture into the pan and cook until the eggs are set.
6. Remove the skillet from heat and serve the scramble.

7. Enjoy.

Nutrition Facts
Servings: 4

Amount per serving

Calories 214

% Daily Value*

Total Fat 14.6g	19%
Saturated Fat 2.7g	14%
Cholesterol 205mg	68%
Sodium 99mg	4%
Total Carbohydrate 12.8g	5%
Dietary Fiber 1.8g	6%
Total Sugars 6g	
Protein 8g	
Vitamin D 19mcg	96%
Calcium 47mg	4%
Iron 1mg	8%
Potassium 261mg	

Eggplant Casserole

PREP TIME: 15 minutes

COOK TIME: 55 minutes

SERVINGS: 8

Ingredients:

- 1 large egg (lightly beaten)
- 1tsp Italian seasoning
- 1 clove garlic (crushed)
- 1 large eggplant (peeled)
- 2 cups plain bread crumbs
- 1 pound lean ground turkey
- 2 tbsp olive oil
- ½ tsp red pepper
- ½ cup green pepper (chopped)
- ½ cup finely chopped onion

Directions:

1. Preheat the oven to 350°F.
2. Place the peeled eggplant in a pot and add enough water.
3. Bring the eggplant and water to a rolling boil and cook until the eggplant is tender.
4. Put the eggplant in a bowl and mash it.
5. Heat up the olive oil in a large skillet over medium to high heat.
6. Add the garlic, onion, green pepper and ground turkey. Saute until the ground turkey is cooked.
7. Add the egg, mashed eggplant and breadcrumbs.

8. Add Italian seasoning and red pepper. Mix until the ingredients are well combined.
9. Pour the mixture in the skillet into a casserole dish.
10. Place the casserole dish in the preheated oven and bake for about 40 to 45 minutes.
11. After the baking cycle, remove the casserole from the oven and let it cool for a few minutes.
12. Serve warm and enjoy

Nutrition Facts
Servings: 8

Amount per serving
Calories 253

% Daily Value*

Total Fat 10g	**13%**
Saturated Fat 2.5g	**13%**
Cholesterol 64mg	**21%**
Sodium 254mg	**11%**
Total Carbohydrate 25.1g	**9%**
Dietary Fiber 3.4g	**12%**
Total Sugars 4.7g	
Protein 16.7g	
Vitamin D 2mcg	11%
Calcium 62mg	5%
Iron 2mg	13%
Potassium 363mg	

Meatloaf (no sauce)

PREP TIME: 15 minutes

COOK TIME: 45 minutes

SERVINGS: 8

Ingredients:

- ½ cup water
- ¼ cup carrots (cooked, drained and finely chopped)
- 2 celery stalks (finely chopped)
- ¼ tsp black pepper
- 1/2tsp onion powder
- ½ cup plain breadcrumbs
- 1 tbsp fresh lemon juice
- ½ tsp Italian seasoning
- ¼ tsp oregano
- Half green pepper (diced)
- 1 small onion (diced)

Directions:

1. Preheat the oven to 400°F and grease loaf pan.
2. Put the ground turkey in a mixing bowl and add the lemon juice. Mix until well combined.
3. Add the diced onion, green pepper, onion powder, black pepper, bread crumbs, carrot, celery and Italian seasoning.
4. Pour water the ingredients in the mixing bowl and mix until the ingredients are well combined.
5. Mold the mixture into a meatloaf and place it in the loaf pan.

6. Place the loaf pan in the preheated oven and bake for about 45 minutes.
7. After the baking cycle, remove the loaf pan and let the meatloaf sit for a few minutes to cool.
8. Cut into slices and serve.

Nutrition Facts	
Servings: 8	
Amount per serving	
Calories	**36**
% Daily Value*	
Total Fat 0.5g	1%
Saturated Fat 0.1g	1%
Cholesterol 0mg	0%
Sodium 57mg	2%
Total Carbohydrate 6.8g	2%
Dietary Fiber 0.8g	3%
Total Sugars 1.3g	
Protein 1.2g	
Vitamin D 0mcg	0%
Calcium 20mg	2%
Iron 0mg	2%
Potassium 67mg	

Renal friendly Lunch, Dinner and Soups

Creamy Celery Soup

PREP TIME: 10 minutes

COOK TIME: 20 minutes

SERVINGS: 8

Ingredients:

- 1 tbsp olive oil
- 4 cups chopped celery
- 2 cups chopped yellow onion
- 1 tsp Italian seasoning
- 1 tbsp freshly chopped thyme
- ¼ tsp salt
- 1 tbsp fresh lemon juice
- 1/2 cup heavy cream
- 1/8 tsp ground black pepper
- 4 cups unsalted chicken broth
- 1 tsp lemon zest
- 1 tsp cumin
- 2 cups fresh baby spinach
- 4 garlic cloves (crushed)
  Garnish:
- 2 tbsp fresh chopped parsley

Directions:

1. Heat up 1 tbsp olive oil in a large pot over medium to high heat.
2. Add the onions, celery, thyme and garlic.
3. Saute for about 10 minutes or until the vegetables are soft, stirring constantly.
4. Stir in the lemon zest, cumin and Italian seasoning.
5. Pour in the chicken broth and add salt.
6. Bring the soup to a boil, reduce the heat and simmer for 6 minutes or until the celery pieces are tender.
7. Add the lemon juice and spinach. Cook for 2 minutes.
8. Remove the pot from heat and use a hand blender to puree the soup until smooth.
9. If you do not have a hand blender, let the soup cool for a few minutes, transfer it to a regular blender and blend until smooth. After blending return the soup to the pot.
10. Stir in the heavy whipping cream and black pepper.
11. Serve soup into bowls and garnish with chopped fresh parsley.
12. Enjoy.

Nutrition Facts

Servings: 8

Amount per serving

Calories 61

% Daily Value*

Total Fat 5g	6%
Saturated Fat 2.1g	10%
Cholesterol 11mg	4%
Sodium 125mg	5%
Total Carbohydrate 3.7g	1%
Dietary Fiber 1.4g	5%
Total Sugars 1.2g	
Protein 1g	
Vitamin D 4mcg	20%
Calcium 48mg	4%
Iron 1mg	6%
Potassium 212mg	

Cucumber Shrimp Soup

PREP TIME: 20 minutes

SERVINGS: 4

Ingredients:

- 1 cup shallot
- ¼ tsp crushed red pepper
- 2 medium cucumber (peeled, seeded and chopped)
- ¼ cup radishes (finely chopped)
- 4 tbsp chopped fresh parsley
- 2 whole garlic cloves (crushed)
- 2 cups unsweetened almond milk
- 3 tbsp fresh lemon juice
- ¼ lemon pepper seasoning
- 8 ounces shrimp (peeled, deveined, cooked and chopped)
- 2 tbsp red wine vinegar
- 1 cup plain fat free Greek yogurt

Directions:

1. Toss the cucumber into a powerful blender and add almond milk, Greek yogurt, lemon juice, crushed red pepper, lemon pepper seasoning, garlic, shallot and parsley. Blend until smooth.
2. Now, the blended mixture into a large mixing bowl.
3. Add the chopped shrimp, vinegar and radishes. Mix until well combined.
4. Place the mixing bowl in a refrigerator and chill the soup for a few minutes.
5. Serve soup into bowls and enjoy.

Nutrition Facts
Servings: 4

Amount per serving
Calories 173

% Daily Value*

Total Fat 3.2g	4%
Saturated Fat 0.6g	3%
Cholesterol 121mg	40%
Sodium 272mg	12%
Total Carbohydrate 14.6g	5%
Dietary Fiber 1.6g	6%
Total Sugars 4.1g	
Protein 21.4g	
Vitamin D 1mcg	3%
Calcium 417mg	32%
Iron 2mg	9%
Potassium 527mg	

Ground beef Soup

PREP TIME: 35 minutes

COOK TIME: 10 minutes

SERVINGS: 6

Ingredients:

- ½ cup onion
- 1tsp allspice
- 1 tbsp fresh lemon juice
- ½ tsp ground black pepper
- 1/3 cup white rice (uncooked)
- 1 tsp hot sauce
- 2 cups water
- 3 cups frozen mixed vegetables (unsalted)
- 1 tbsp sour cream
- 1 cup low sodium beef broth

Directions:

1. Heat up a large saucepan over medium to high heat.
2. Add the onion ground beef and saute until the ground beef and onion are browned, stirring often. Drain the beef fat.
3. Pour in the water and add the allspice, lemon juice, pepper, hot sauce, mixed vegetables, broth and rice.
4. Bring the soup to a boil, cover the saucepan, reduce the heat and simmer the soup for30 minutes.
5. Remove the saucepan from heat and stir in the sour cream.
6. Serve and enjoy.

Nutrition Facts
Servings: 6

Amount per serving
Calories 113

% Daily Value*

Total Fat 0.9g	1%
Saturated Fat 0.4g	2%
Cholesterol 1mg	0%
Sodium 185mg	8%
Total Carbohydrate 21.7g	8%
Dietary Fiber 4.5g	**16%**
Total Sugars 3.4g	
Protein 4.4g	
Vitamin D 0mcg	0%
Calcium 37mg	3%
Iron 1mg	8%
Potassium 228mg	

Vegetable Soup

PREP TIME: 15 minutes

COOK TIME: 50 minutes

SERVINGS: 5

Ingredients:

- 2tbsp olive oil
- 1tsp oregano
- 1tsp garlic powder
- 1 tsp thyme
- ½ tsp curry
- ¼ tsp coriander
- ¼ tsp salt
- 4 cups low sodium vegetable broth
- 1/2cup frozen corn
- 1 cup fresh green beans
- ¾ cup celery
- ½ cup onion
- ½ cup carrots (diced)
- 1 small tomato (diced)
- ½ cup mushrooms (chopped)

Directions:

1. Heat up the olive oil in a large pot over medium to high heat.
2. Add the onion and celery and saute the onion is soft and lightly browned.
3. Add the carrots, tomato, mushrooms, corn and green beans.
4. Pour in the vegetable broth and add the salt, curry, thyme, garlic powder, oregano and coriander.

5. Bring the soup to a boil, reduce the heat to medium-low and simmer the soup for about 45 to 50 minutes.
6. Remove the pot from heat and let the soup cool for a few minutes.
7. Serve warm and enjoy.

Nutrition Facts
Servings: 5

Amount per serving
Calories 100

% **Daily Value***

Total Fat 6g	8%
Saturated Fat 0.9g	4%
Cholesterol 0mg	0%
Sodium 454mg	20%
Total Carbohydrate 12.1g	4%
Dietary Fiber 2.6g	9%
Total Sugars 3.6g	
Protein 1.8g	
Vitamin D 25mcg	126%
Calcium 32mg	2%
Iron 1mg	8%
Potassium 260mg	

Pumpkin Chili

PREP TIME: 10 minutes

COOK TIME: 1 hour 10minutes

SERVINGS: 10

Ingredients:

- 2 tbsp olive oil
- 2 pound ground turkey breast
- ½ cup onion (finely chopped)
- ½ cup carrots (finely chopped)
- 1 tsp oregano
- 1tsp ground black pepper
- 1 tsp allspice
- 1 tbsp chili powder
- ½ cup canned unsalted green chiles (chopped)
- ½ cup red kidney beans
- 2 garlic cloves (crushed)
- 12 ounces canned pumpkin puree
- 2 tsp cumin
- 3 cups low sodium chicken broth
- 2 bay leaves
- 1 tsp thyme

Directions:

1. Heat up one tbsp olive oil in a large pot over medium to high heat.
2. Add the garlic, onion, carrot and celery and saute until the vegetables are tender, stirring often.

3. Use a slotted spoon to transfer the roasted vegetables to a clean plate.
4. Add the remaining olive oil and the ground turkey. Break the ground turkey apart and saute until it is browned.
5. Pour in the chicken broth to deglaze the pot.
6. Add the roasted vegetables, thyme, bay leaves, black pepper, chili, pumpkin puree, green chiles, kidney beans, oregano, cumin and allspice.
7. Bring the soup to a boil, reduce the heat and simmer the soup for an hour, stirring occasionally.
8. Remove the pot from heat and discard the bay leaves.
9. Serve soup into bowls and enjoy.

Nutrition Facts
Servings: 10

Amount per serving
Calories 256

% Daily Value*

Total Fat 10g	13%
Saturated Fat 2.4g	12%
Cholesterol 67mg	22%
Sodium 139mg	6%
Total Carbohydrate 11.5g	4%
Dietary Fiber 3.2g	11%
Total Sugars 2.3g	
Protein 29.5g	
Vitamin D 0mcg	0%
Calcium 53mg	4%
Iron 3mg	19%
Potassium 515mg	

Rotisserie Chicken

PREP TIME: 15 minutes

COOK TIME: 2 hours 30 minutes

SERVINGS: 8

Ingredients:

- 4 pound whole chicken
- 1 tsp pepper
- ¼ tsp salt
- 1 tsp Italian seasoning
- 2 tsp dried Greek seasoning
- 1 large red onion (halved)
- 2 tbsp olive oil
- ½ tsp paprika

Directions:

1. Preheat the oven to 300°F.
2. In small bowl, combine all the salt, pepper, Italian seasoning, paprika and dried Greek seasoning.
3. Divide the mixed ingredient into three.
4. Use your fingers to loosen the skin from the chicken breast.
5. Rub 1 tbsp olive oil and 1/3 of the seasoning under the chicken skin.
6. Rub 1 tbsp olive oil and 2/3 of the seasoning all over the chicken body; deep your hand into the chicken and rub the oil and seasoning into the body cavity as well.
7. Insert the halved onion into the chicken body cavity.
8. Pour 1 cup of water into the button of a roasting pan and place a roasting rack in the pan.
9. Place the chicken on the roasting rack, chest side down.

10. Place the roasting pan in the oven and bake for about 2 hours 30 minutes or until a meat thermometer inserted into the inner thigh reads 160°F.
11. Remove the roasting pan from the oven and leave the chicken to cool for about 15 minutes.
12. Cut into sizes and serve.

Nutrition Facts
Servings: 8

Amount per serving
Calories   473

% Daily Value*

Total Fat 20.6g	**26%**
Saturated Fat 5.2g	**26%**
Cholesterol 202mg	**67%**
Sodium 309mg	**13%**
Total Carbohydrate 2.4g	**1%**
Dietary Fiber 0.5g	**2%**
Total Sugars 0.9g	
Protein 65.9g	
Vitamin D 0mcg	0%
Calcium 40mg	3%
Iron 3mg	16%
Potassium 590mg	

Barley Soup

PREP TIME: 15 minutes

COOK TIME: 2 hours 10 minutes

SERVINGS: 6

Ingredients:

- 1 pound lean beef (cut into 1 inch cubes)
- ¼ tsp salt
- 2 quarts water
- ¼ cup chopped carrot
- 1 garlic clove(minced)
- 1 cup raw pearl barley (soaked and drained)
- ½ cup onion (chopped)
- ¼ tsp black pepper
- 2 tbsp all-purpose flour
- 2 stalk celery (chopped)
- 2bay leaves
- 1tsp paprika
- 1 tsp cumin
- 1 tsp dried basil
- 2 tbsp olive oil

Directions:

1. In a mixing bowl, mix the black pepper and all-purpose flour. Add the beef cubes and toss until they are coated with the flour mixture.
2. Heat up the olive oil in a heavy pot over medium to high heat.

3. Add the meat and saute until it is browned, turning occasionally.
4. Use a slotted spoon to transfer the browned beef to a paper towel lined plate.
5. Add the onion, celery and garlic. Saute until the vegetables are tender.
6. Add water and bring the mixture to a boil.
7. Add the browned meat, bay leaves, barley salt. Reduce heat and simmer for an hour, stirring occasionally.
8. Add carrots, basil, cumin and paprika. Cover and simmer for another 1 hour.
9. Remove the pot from heat and discard the bay leaves.
10. Serve the soup into bowl and enjoy.

Nutrition Facts
Servings: 6

Amount per serving	
Calories	**318**
	% Daily Value*
Total Fat 10g	13%
Saturated Fat 2.6g	13%
Cholesterol 68mg	23%
Sodium 168mg	7%
Total Carbohydrate 30.1g	11%
Dietary Fiber 5.9g	21%
Total Sugars 1.1g	
Protein 26.9g	

Nutrition Facts
Servings: 6

Vitamin D 0mcg	0%
Calcium 34mg	3%
Iron 16mg	87%
Potassium 466mg	

Chicken noodle soup

PREP TIME: 10 minutes

COOK TIME: 50 minutes

SERVINGS: 8

Ingredients:

- ½ cup chopped green pepper
- 1 cup egg noodles
- 1 tsp sugar
- 2 celery stalks (chopped)
- 3 tbsp fresh lemon juice
- 2 tbsp olive oil
- 1 tbsp poultry dressing
- 1 pound chicken thigh
- 1 tsp oregano
- 1 tsp ground black pepper
- 1 tsp dried basil
- 1 tsp crushed red pepper
- 3 ½ cups water
- ½ onion (chopped)
- 2 clove garlic (minced)

Directions:

1. Heat up the olive oil in a large pot over medium to high heat.
2. Add the onion, green pepper, celery and garlic. Saute until the vegetables are tender.
3. Pour in the water and add the chicken, lemon juice, black pepper, red pepper, basil, oregano and sugar. Bring to a

boil, reduce the heat and simmer the soup for 30 minutes or until the chicken is soft.
4. Add the egg noodles and cook for 15 minutes. Add more water if the soup is too thick.
5. Remove the pot from heat and serve the soup into bowls.

Nutrition Facts
Servings: 8

Amount per serving	
Calories	176
	% Daily Value*
Total Fat 8.3g	11%
Saturated Fat 1.8g	9%
Cholesterol 56mg	19%
Sodium 58mg	3%
Total Carbohydrate 7.2g	3%
Dietary Fiber 0.8g	3%
Total Sugars 1.2g	
Protein 17.6g	
Vitamin D 0mcg	0%
Calcium 24mg	2%
Iron 1mg	6%
Potassium 198mg	

Chicken Rice Soup

PREP TIME: 15 minutes

COOK TIME: 28 minutes

SERVINGS: 8

Ingredients:

- 2 boneless skinless chicken breast (cut into small bite sizes)
- 10 cups low sodium chicken broth
- 1 tsp paprika
- 1 bay leaf
- 1 cup chopped carrots
- 1 cup chopped celery
- 1 tsp ground black pepper
- ¾ cups white rice (uncooked)
- 1 tsp thyme
- 1 cup chopped onions
- 1 tsp garlic powder
- 1 tsp mustard
  Garnish:
- 3 tbsp fresh chopped parsley
- 2 tbsp fresh lemon juice

Directions:

1. In a large heavy pot, combine the rice, onion, celery, carrots, bay leaf, thyme, garlic powder, mustard, black pepper and paprika.

2. Pour in the chicken broth and bring the mixture to a boil. Cover the pot, reduce heat and simmer soup for about 20 minutes.
3. Add the chicken pieces and cook for 5 to 8 minutes or until the chicken pieces are tender.
4. Remove the pot from heat and discard the bay leaves.
5. Stir in the lemon juice and chopped fresh parsley. Serve and enjoy.

Nutrition Facts

Servings: 8

Amount per serving

Calories 137

% **Daily Value***

Total Fat 1.4g	2%
Saturated Fat 0.5g	2%
Cholesterol 16mg	5%
Sodium 120mg	5%
Total Carbohydrate 19.2g	7%
Dietary Fiber 1.5g	5%
Total Sugars 1.7g	
Protein 10.7g	
Vitamin D 0mcg	0%
Calcium 27mg	2%
Iron 2mg	11%
Potassium 148mg	

Meatball Soup

PREP TIME: 20 minutes

COOK TIME: 45 minutes

SERVINGS: 12

Ingredients:

- 1 ½ pound lean ground beef
- 3 cups low sodium beef broth
- 3 cups water
- 1 tsp ground cumin
- ½ tsp garlic powder
- 1 tsp Italian seasoning
- ½ cup fresh spinach (chopped)
- 2 garlic cloves (chopped)
- 1 large onion (chopped)
- 1 cup uncooked white rice
- 1 medium roma tomato (finely chopped)
- 1 tsp black pepper
- 2 tbsp chopped red bell pepper
- 2 tbsp freshly chopped parsley
- 1 tbsp lime juice
  Garnish:
- 2 tbsp chopped fresh cilantro (optional)

Directions:

1. In a mixing bowl, combine the ground beef, parsley, lemon juice, cumin and garlic powder.
2. Mold the mixture into meatballs and arrange the meatballs into a large pot.

3. Add the water and beef broth.
4. Bring to a boil and reduce the heat.
5. Add the chopped onion, Italian seasoning, red bell pepper, black pepper, tomato and chopped garlic.
6. Cover the pot and simmer the soup for 40 minutes.
7. Stir in the chopped spinach and cook for 5 minutes more.
8. Remove pot from heat and stir in the chopped fresh cilantro.
9. Serve and enjoy.

Nutrition Facts
Servings: 12

Amount per serving
Calories 188

% Daily Value*

Total Fat 4.2g	5%
Saturated Fat 1.5g	7%
Cholesterol 51mg	17%
Sodium 234mg	10%
Total Carbohydrate 16.2g	6%
Dietary Fiber 1g	3%
Total Sugars 2g	
Protein 20.1g	
Vitamin D 0mcg	0%
Calcium 20mg	2%
Iron 12mg	66%
Potassium 387mg	

Cauliflower Soup

PREP TIME: 20 minutes

COOK TIME: 30 minutes

SERVINGS: 6

Ingredients:

- 2 tbsp olive oil
- 2 celery stalks (chopped)
- 2 small carrots (finely chopped)
- 2 garlic cloves (minced)
- 1 small onion (chopped)
- 3 cups water
- 1 small head cauliflower (cut into florets)
- ½ cup light sour cream
- 2 tsp curry powder
- 2 tbsp chopped fresh parsley
- ½ tsp paprika

Directions:

1. Heat up the olive oil in a large saucepan over medium to high heat.
2. Add the onion, celery, garlic and carrot. Saute for 4 to 5 minutes or until the vegetables are tender, stirring often.
3. Pour in the water and add cauliflower, curry and paprika.
4. Bring to a boil, reduce the heat and simmer the soup for about 20 minutes or until the cauliflower is softened.
5. Remove the pot from heat and puree the soup with an immersion blender until smooth.

6. If you do not have and immersion blender, let the soup cool a bit, transfer it into a food processor and blend until smooth. After blending, transfer the soup to the saucepan.
7. Return the soup to heat and stir in the sour cream and chopped fresh parsley.
8. Cook the soup for 4 minutes.
9. Remove the soup from heat and serve the soup into bowls.

Nutrition Facts
Servings: 6

Amount per serving
Calories 109

% Daily Value*

Total Fat 8.9g **11%**

Saturated Fat 3.2g **16%**

Cholesterol 8mg **3%**

Sodium 45mg **2%**

Total Carbohydrate 7g **3%**

Dietary Fiber 2.2g **8%**

Total Sugars 2.5g

Protein 2g

Vitamin D 0mcg 0%

Calcium 53mg 4%

Iron 1mg 3%

Potassium 273mg

Cabbage Stew

PREP TIME: 18 minutes

COOK TIME: 35 minutes

SERVINGS: 6

Ingredients:

- 1 tbsp olive oil
- 1 tsp oregano
- 1 tbsp chopped fresh thyme
- 1 tsp chopped savory
- 2 tbsp fresh chopped cilantro
- 1 green onion (chopped)
- 1 sweet onion (chopped)
- 2 celery stalks (chopped)
- 2 tbsp fresh lemon juice
- 1 tsp ground black pepper
- 1 bay leaf
- 6 cups shredded cabbage
- 2 garlic cloves (minced)
- 1 cup fresh green beans (chopped)
- Water (as needed)

Directions:

1. Heat up the olive oil in a Dutch oven over medium to high heat.
2. Add the onion, celery and garlic. Saute for about 4 minutes or until the vegetables are tender.

3. Add the cabbage, lemon juice, savory, thyme, parsley, green onion, oregano, black pepper and bay leaf. Stir and add enough water.
4. Bring the soup to a boil, reduce the heat to medium low and simmer the soup for 25 minutes or until the vegetables are tender.
5. Stir in the green beans and cook for additional 3 minutes.
6. Remove the stew from heat and discard the bay leave.
7. Serve into bowls and enjoy.

Nutrition Facts

Servings: 6

Amount per serving

Calories 59

% Daily Value*

Total Fat 2.6g	**3%**
Saturated Fat 0.4g	**2%**
Cholesterol 0mg	**0%**
Sodium 21mg	**1%**
Total Carbohydrate 8.8g	**3%**
Dietary Fiber 3.5g	**12%**
Total Sugars 3.6g	
Protein 1.8g	
Vitamin D 0mcg	0%
Calcium 65mg	5%
Iron 2mg	9%
Potassium 233mg	

Cucumber Salad

PREP TIME: 15 minutes

SERVINGS: 4

Ingredients:

- 1 large raw cucumber (peeled and sliced)
- 300 g mixed salad greens
- 2 medium apple (peeled and cubed)
- 1 large carrot (peeled and sliced)
- ½ cup sugar
- 2/3 cup rice vinegar
- 1 cup fresh pineapple cubes
- 1/3 cup chopped sweet onion
- 1 tsp mustard
- 1 tbsp toasted sesame seeds

Directions:

1. Combine the sugar, rice vinegar, mustard and paprika in a saucepan over heat. Bring to a boil and cook for about 5 minutes, stirring constantly.
2. Pour the mixture into a large mixing bowl, cover the bowl and place it in a refrigerator. Refrigerate for about 15 minutes.
3. Remove the mixing bowl from the fridge and add the pineapple and apple.
4. Return the mixing bowl to the refrigerator and refrigerate for 1 hour.
5. Bring out the mixing bowl and add the cucumber, onion and carrot. Toss to combine.

6. Serve with salad greens and garnish with toasted sesame seeds.

Nutrition Facts
Servings: 4

Amount per serving
Calories 160

% Daily Value*

Total Fat 1.9g	**2%**
Saturated Fat 0.2g	**1%**
Cholesterol 0mg	**0%**
Sodium 33mg	**1%**
Total Carbohydrate 30.6g	**11%**
Dietary Fiber 2.5g	**9%**
Total Sugars 22.1g	
Protein 1.6g	

Vitamin D 0mcg	0%
Calcium 51mg	4%
Iron 1mg	4%
Potassium 257mg	

Shrimp Scampi

PREP TIME: 5 minutes

COOK TIME: 5 minutes

SERVINGS: 4

Ingredients:

- 1 ¼ pound large shrimp (peeled and deveined)
- 1 medium onion (finely chopped)
- 1 roma tomatoes (thinly sliced)
- 1 tsp ground black pepper
- ¼ tsp crushed red bell pepper flakes
- 1 tsp salt
- 4 tbsp butter
- 2 tbsp olive oil
- 2 garlic cloves (grated)
- ¼ cup dry white wine
- 2 tbsp fresh lemon juice
- 3 tbsp chopped fresh parsley

Directions:

1. Heat up the olive oil and butter in a large skillet over medium to high heat.
2. Add the onion, garlic and tomato and stir cook for about 2 minutes.
3. Stir in the white wine, crush red pepper flakes, ground black pepper and salt.
4. Bring to a boil and simmer for about 2 to 3 minutes or until the liquid content has reduces by half.

5. Add the shrimp and cook until they are just pink. This will take about 3 to 4 minutes.
6. Stir in the lemon juice and chopped parsley. Remove the skillet from heat.
7. Serve over rice or pasta and enjoy.

Nutrition Facts
Servings: 4

Amount per serving
Calories 311

% Daily Value*

Total Fat 18.7g	**24%**
Saturated Fat 8.4g	**42%**
Cholesterol 233mg	**78%**
Sodium 266mg	**12%**
Total Carbohydrate 7.9g	**3%**
Dietary Fiber 1.3g	**4%**
Total Sugars 2.3g	
Protein 27.6g	
Vitamin D 8mcg	40%
Calcium 24mg	2%
Iron 1mg	3%
Potassium 169mg	

Kidney Friendly Pizza

PREP TIME: 30 minutes

COOK TIME: 30 minutes

SERVINGS: 10 (10 slices)

Ingredients:

Pizza sauce ingredients:

- 1 tsp olive oil
- ½ cup water
- 1 pound lean ground chicken
- ½ tsp Italian seasoning
- 1 tsp chili powder
- 1 tsp paprika
- 1/2tsp garlic powder
- ½ tsp onion powder
- ½ cup tomato paste
- 1 green bell pepper (finely chopped)
- 1 large onion (diced)
- 4 ounces grated low fat sharp cheddar cheese (divided)

Pizza Crust Ingredients:

- 1 tsp cinnamon
- 1 cup warm water (45° F)
- 2 tbsp vegetable shortening
- 1 tsp active dry yeast
- 1 tbsp granulated sugar
- 2 cups all-purpose flour

Directions:

1. In a large mixing bowl, combine the all-purpose flour, cinnamon, yeast and sugar. Add the vegetable shortening and mix.
2. Mix the ingredients until you form smooth dough, adding warm water in bit while mixing.
3. Cover the dough and let it sit for 15 minutes to rise.
4. Meanwhile, preheat the oven to 425°F and start making the pizza sauce.
5. Heat up the olive oil in a pan over medium to high heat.
6. Add the ground chicken and saute until it is browned.
7. Use a slotted spoon to transfer the chicken to a paper towel lined plated to drain. Discard the cooking fat.
8. In a mixing bowl, combine the tomato paste, water paprika, chili powder and Italian seasoning.
9. Grease a pizza pan and spread the pizza dough into the pan.
10. Pour in the tomato paste mixture over the pizza dough and sprinkle half of the cheese over the tomato paste mixture.
11. Place the pizza pan in the preheated oven and bake for 17 to 20 minutes.
12. Remove the pan from the oven and add the beef, green pepper and chopped onion.
13. Sprinkle the remaining cheese over the pizza.
14. Return the pizza pan to the oven and bake for 10 minutes.
15. After the baking cycle, remove the pizza from the oven and let it sit for a few minutes.
16. Slice into sizes and serve.

Nutrition Facts
Servings: 10

Amount per serving
Calories 236

% Daily Value*

Total Fat 7.8g	**10%**
Saturated Fat 2.9g	**15%**
Cholesterol 38mg	**13%**
Sodium 137mg	**6%**
Total Carbohydrate 25.9g	**9%**
Dietary Fiber 2.1g	**7%**
Total Sugars 4.2g	
Protein 16.1g	
Vitamin D 0mcg	0%
Calcium 99mg	8%
Iron 2mg	12%
Potassium 226mg	

Irish stew

PREP TIME: 20 minutes

COOK TIME: 1 hour 5 minutes

SERVINGS: 4

Ingredients:

- 1 tbsp olive oil
- 10 ounces beef (cubed)
- 1 tsp chopped parsley
- ¼ tsp black pepper
- ¼ tsp oregano
- ½ tsp rosemary
- ½ tsp savory
- 1 garlic clove (crushed)
- 1 cup potato (cubed)*see notes
- 1 large onion (chopped)
- ½ cup chopped carrots (boiled, drained and rinsed)
- 1 ½ cup low sodium beef broth

Directions:

1. Put the potato pieces in a pot and add enough water.
2. Bring the water and potato to a boil.
3. Drain off the hot water and add fresh water.
4. Bring the fresh water and potatoes to a boil and cook until the potato pieces are tender.
5. Drain the water and set aside.
6. Heat up the olive oil in a pot and add the beef cubes. Saute until the beef cubes are browned, turning occasionally.

7. Use a perforated spoon to transfer the beef to a paper towel lined plate.
8. Add the onion and garlic to the oil in the pot and saute until the vegetables are tender, stirring constantly.
9. Pour in the beef broth and add the savory, rosemary, oregano, black pepper and parsley.
10. Bring soup to a boil, reduce the heat, cover the pot and simmer the stew for an hour.
11. Add the carrots and potatoes and cook for additional 5 minutes.
12. Remove the pot from heat and serve the soup into bowls.

Note: double boiling the potatoes according to the directions given help to reduce the potassium content of the potato.

Nutrition Facts
Servings: 4

Amount per serving
Calories 222

% Daily Value*

Total Fat 8.5g — 11%
  Saturated Fat 2.3g — 12%
Cholesterol 63mg — 21%
Sodium 346mg — 15%
Total Carbohydrate 10.8g — 4%
  Dietary Fiber 2g — 7%
  Total Sugars 2.8g
Protein 24.5g

Vitamin D 0mcg — 0%
Calcium 31mg — 2%
Iron 14mg — 78%
Potassium 594mg

Turkey Stuffed Pepper

PREP TIME: 15 minutes

COOK TIME: 30 minutes

SERVINGS: 6

Ingredients:

- 6 medium green peppers
- ½ pound ground lean turkey
- 2 tbsp olive oil
- 1 tbsp celery seeds
- 1 tsp black ground pepper
- 1 ½ cups cooked white rice
- 1 tsp sugar
- 2 tbsp Italian seasoning
- 2 tbsp fresh lemon juice
- 1 small onion (chopped)
- 2 stalk celery (chopped)
- 1 tsp paprika
- 2 tsp chopped parsley

Directions:

1. Preheat the oven to 325°F and line a baking dish with parchment paper.
2. Cut off the top of the green peppers pepper and remove the seeds. Set aside.
3. Heat up the olive oil in a saucepan over medium to high heat.
4. Add the ground turkey, celery and onion and saute until the turkey is browned, stirring often.

5. Stir in the paprika, sugar, celery seed, Italian seasoning, parsley, pepper, lemon juice and cooked rice. Remove the saucepan from heat.
6. Fill the green peppers with equal amount of the mixture and arrange the stuffed pepper into the baking dish.
7. Cover the baking dish and place it in the preheated oven.
8. Bake for 30 minutes.
9. Remove the baking dish from the oven, uncover it and let the stuffed peppers cool for a few minutes.
10. Serve warm and enjoy.

Nutrition Facts
Servings: 6

Amount per serving
Calories 312

% Daily Value*

Total Fat 9.3g	**12%**
Saturated Fat 1.1g	**6%**
Cholesterol 25mg	**8%**
Sodium 42mg	**2%**
Total Carbohydrate 45.7g	**17%**
Dietary Fiber 3.3g	**12%**
Total Sugars 4.7g	
Protein 12.2g	
Vitamin D 0mcg	0%
Calcium 51mg	4%
Iron 3mg	18%
Potassium 328mg	

Orange Chicken

PREP TIME: 2 hours 20 minutes

COOK TIME: 20 minutes

SERVINGS: 4

Ingredients:

- 3 tbsp olive oil
- 354 ml (1 ½ cup) water
- ½ pound boneless skinless chicken breast (cut into small bite sizes)
- 1 garlic clove (minced)
- 2 tbsp fresh orange juice
- ½ tsp ground black pepper
- ¼ tsp paprika
- 2 tbsp chopped green onion
- ½ tsp ginger powder
- ¼ cup fresh lemon juice
- 2 ½ tsp cornstarch + 4 tbsp water for mixing
- 2 tbsp low sodium soy sauce
- 1/3 cup organic rice vinegar
- 1/3 cup brown sugar
  Garnish:
- 2 tbsp chopped fresh parsley

Directions:

1. In a large saucepan, combine the water, soy sauce, rice vinegar, orange juice, lemon juice, brown sugar, green onion, pepper, paprika, garlic, ginger, over medium to high heat.

2. Bring the mixture to a boil. Remove pot from and let the sauce cool for about 12 minutes.
3. Put the chicken pieces in a large mixing bowl and pour 1 cup of the sauce over it. Stir to combine.
4. Cover the mixing bowl and place it in a refrigerator. Marinate for 2 hours.
5. Heat up the olive oil in a large skillet over medium to high heat.
6. Add the marinated chicken and saute until the chicken pieces are browned.
7. Use a slotted spoon to transfer the browned chicken to a paper towel lined plate. Discard the cooking oil and wipe the skillet clean.
8. Pour the remaining sauce into the skillet and bring to a boil over medium to high heat.
9. Mix the cornstarch with 4 tbsp water in a small bowl. Add the mixed cornstarch to the sauce and reduce heat.
10. Add the browned chicken and cook for 5 minutes, stirring occasionally.
11. Remove the sauce from heat.
12. Serve the orange chicken into bowls and garnish with chopped fresh parsley.

Nutrition Facts

Servings: 4

Amount per serving

Calories 280

% Daily Value*

Total Fat 14.9g	**19%**
Saturated Fat 2.8g	**14%**
Cholesterol 50mg	**17%**
Sodium 357mg	**16%**
Total Carbohydrate 16.3g	**6%**
Dietary Fiber 0.5g	**2%**
Total Sugars 13g	
Protein 17.3g	
Vitamin D 0mcg	0%
Calcium 29mg	2%
Iron 1mg	8%
Potassium 236mg	

Indian Chickpea Curry (Chana Masala)

PREP TIME: 10 minutes

COOK TIME: 25 minutes

SERVINGS: 4

Ingredients:

- 30 ounces canned lower sodium chickpeas (rinsed and drained) Trader Joe®
- 2 tbsp olive oil
- ½ cup water
- 8 ounce canned diced tomatoes (unsalted)
- 3 garlic cloves (minced)
- 1 tsp garam masala
- 1 tsp ground turmeric
- 1 tsp coriander
- 1 tsp chili powder
- 1 tsp allspice
- ½ tsp paprika
- 1 small onion (chopped)
- 1 stalk of small celery (chopped)
- ½ tsp ginger powder
  Garnish:
- 2 tbsp chopped parsley
- 4 lemon wedges

Directions:

1. Heat up the olive oil over medium to high heat.
2. Add the onion, celery and garlic. Saute for about 3 minutes or until the vegetables are tender.

3. Add the diced tomatoes and cook for 4 minutes.
4. Stir in the garam masala, paprika, allspice, turmeric, chili powder, coriander and ginger powder. Cook for 1 minute.
5. Pour in the water and add the chickpeas.
6. Reduce the heat and simmer the chickpea curry for about 15 minutes.
7. Remove the skillet from heat and serve into bowl.
8. Garnish chopped parsley and lemon wedges.

Nutrition Facts

Servings: 4

Amount per serving

Calories 295

% Daily Value*

Total Fat 9.1g	**12%**
Saturated Fat 1.1g	5%
Cholesterol 0mg	**0%**
Sodium 392mg	**17%**
Total Carbohydrate 44.3g	**16%**
Dietary Fiber 2g	7%
Total Sugars 12.8g	
Protein 11.4g	
Vitamin D 0mcg	0%
Calcium 31mg	2%
Iron 11mg	62%
Potassium 241mg	

Tofu Stir Fry with Rice

PREP TIME: 15 minutes

COOK TIME: 15 minutes

SERVINGS: 4

Ingredients:

- 1 tbsp + 1 tsp olive oil
- 2 cups steamed white rice
- 16 ounces extra firm tofu (cut into 1 inch cubes)
- 2 tsp sugar
- ¼ chopped red bell pepper
- ½ cup plain bread crumbs
- 1 ½ tbsp lime juice
- ¼ tsp garlic powder
- 2 tbsp cornstarch
- 1 tbsp low sodium sauce
- 1/8 tsp black pepper
- 1/8 tsp cayenne pepper
- ½ tsp allspice
- ½ tsp ground cumin
- 2 egg whites
- 1 cup broccoli (roughly chopped)
  Garnish:
- 1 tsp sesame seed

Directions:

1. Put the egg whites, breadcrumbs and cornstarch into 3 different bowls.

2. Dip each tofu cube into the cornstarch, and then the egg and finally the breadcrumbs. Arrange the coated tofu cubes into a separate plate.
3. Heat up 1 tbsp olive oil in a large skillet. Add the coated tofu cubes and fry until the cubes are browned, stirring often.
4. Use slotted spoon to transfer the browned tofu to a paper towel lined plate.
5. In a mixing bowl, combine the soy sauce, sugar and lime juice. Set aside
6. Add the remaining 1 tsp olive oil to the skillet. Add the chopped broccoli florets and red pepper. Saute until tender and crispy, stirring often.
7. Stir in the allspice, cumin, cayenne, black pepper and garlic.
8. Add the browned tofu cubes. Stir to combine.
9. Stir in the sauce mixture and cook for additional 1 minute.
10. Remove the skillet from heat and stir in the sesame seed.
11. Serve over steamed rice and enjoy.

Nutrition Facts
Servings: 4

Amount per serving
Calories 554

% Daily Value*

Total Fat 10.2g — **13%**

  Saturated Fat 2g — **10%**

Cholesterol 0mg — **0%**

Sodium 294mg — **13%**

Total Carbohydrate 95.2g **35%**

  Dietary Fiber 3.7g — **13%**

  Total Sugars 4.9g

Protein 20.9g

Vitamin D 0mcg — 0%

Calcium 300mg — 23%

Iron 7mg — 39%

Potassium 416mg

Chicken Salad

PREP TIME: 15 minutes

SERVINGS: 4

Ingredients:

- 1 tsp sesame oil
- 1 ½ cup cooked chicken
- A pinch of oregano
- 1 medium apple(peeled and cubed)
- 1 tsp dried parsley
- ¼ tsp cracked black pepper
- 1 tbsp fresh lime juice
- 1 small sweet onion (chopped)
- 1 medium bell pepper (chopped)
- 2 stalk celery (diced)
- ¼ cup radishes (chopped)
- 1 tsp dry mustard
- ½ tsp dried tarragon

Directions:

1. In a small mixing bowl, combine the mustard, mayonnaise, black pepper, oregano and tarragon.
2. Put the chicken into a large mixing bowl and add the onion, radishes, parsley, green pepper and lemon juice. Toss until well combined.
3. Pour the mayonnaise mixture over the chicken and veggies. Toss until well combined.
4. Cover the bowl and chill the salad in a refrigerator.
5. Serve into bowls and drizzle with sesame oil.

Nutrition Facts
Servings: 4

Amount per serving
Calories 143

% Daily Value*

Total Fat 3.2g	**4%**
Saturated Fat 0.6g	**3%**
Cholesterol 40mg	**13%**
Sodium 45mg	**2%**
Total Carbohydrate 12.8g	**5%**
Dietary Fiber 2.6g	**9%**
Total Sugars 8.4g	
Protein 16.2g	
Vitamin D 0mcg	0%
Calcium 26mg	2%
Iron 1mg	6%
Potassium 295mg	

Renal Friendly Snacks, Side Dishes, Desserts and Appetizers

Energy Balls

PREP TIME: 25 minutes

SERVINGS: 20 Balls

Ingredients:

- ½ cup roasted almonds
- 2 tsp cinnamon
- 1 tbsp maple syrup
- 4 tbsp almond butter
- ¼ tsp salt
- ½ cup pitted Medjool dates
- ½ cup coconut flakes

Directions:

1. Toss the almond and date into a blender and blitz until smooth.
2. Add the almond butter, maple syrup, cinnamon and salt.
3. Blend until the ingredients are well combined and smooth.
4. Put the mixture in a bowl, cover the bowl and place it in a refrigerator.
5. Chill for about 10 minutes or until the mixture is firmer.
6. Put the coconut flakes in a bowl.
7. Scoop out equal amount of the mixture with a spoon and mold into balls.

8. Deep each ball into the coconut flakes and arrange them into a parchment paper lined cookie sheet.
9. Serve and enjoy.

Nutrition Facts

Servings: 20

Amount per serving

Calories 55

% Daily Value*

Total Fat 3.7g	5%
Saturated Fat 0.8g	4%
Cholesterol 0mg	0%
Sodium 32mg	1%
Total Carbohydrate 5.3g	2%
Dietary Fiber 1.3g	5%
Total Sugars 3.1g	
Protein 1.4g	
Vitamin D 0mcg	0%
Calcium 12mg	1%
Iron 1mg	6%
Potassium 78mg	

Roasted Chickpea Snack

PREP TIME: 5 minutes

COOK TIME: 20 minutes

SERVINGS: 4

Ingredients:

- 15 ounce canned lower sodium chickpea (drained and rinsed) Trader Joe®
- ½ tsp dried thyme
- 1 tbsp extra virgin olive oil
- ¼ teaspoon freshly ground black pepper
- ½ teaspoon ground cumin
- ½ teaspoon smoked paprika
- ½ teaspoon onion powder
- ½ teaspoon garlic powder
- ½ teaspoon ground coriander

Directions:

1. Preheat the oven to 400°F.
2. Pat the chickpeas dry with paper towel.
3. Spray a baking sheet with nonstick spray and spread the chickpeas on the baking sheet.
4. Place the baking sheet in the preheated oven and bake for 15 minutes
5. Meanwhile, combine the salt, garlic powder, coriander, paprika, black pepper, onion powder, cumin and thyme in a mixing bowl.
6. Remove the baking sheet from the oven.

7. Drizzle oil over the chickpeas and toss until the chickpeas are coated with oil.
8. Add the mixed ingredients and toss until the chickpeas are all coated.
9. Return the chickpeas to the oven and bake for 10 minutes.
10. Remove the baking sheet from the oven and stir the chickpeas.
11. Return the chickpeas to the oven and bake for another 10 minutes.
12. Remove the baking sheet from the oven and allow the chickpeas to cool for a few minutes.
13. Serve and enjoy.

Nutritional Facts:

Per serving: 161 calories; 4.8 g total fat (0.6 g saturated fat); 0 mg cholesterol; 377 mg sodium; 203 mg potassium; 25 g carbohydrates; 4.9 g dietary fiber; 0.2 g sugars; 5.5 g protein

Roasted Brussels sprouts and Bacon

PREP TIME: 15 minutes

COOK TIME: 25 minutes

SERVINGS: 6

Ingredients:

- 1 ½ pounds Brussels sprouts (washed, dried and halved)
- 1 medium red onion (finely chopped)
- 4 ounce diced raw bacon
- 2 tbsp olive oil
- 6 garlic cloves (finely chopped)
- 1 tsp ground black pepper

Directions:

1. Preheat the oven to 220°C and line a large baking pan with aluminum foil.
2. Place the onions, Brussels sprouts, garlic and bacon in the baking pan.
3. Drizzle the ingredients with olive oil and season with salt and pepper.
4. Toss until the ingredients are well combined.
5. Spread out the ingredients in a single layer.
6. Place the baking pan in the preheated oven and bake for about 25 to 30 minutes, turning halfway.
7. After the baking cycle, remove the baking pan from the oven and leave the sprouts and bacon to cool for a few minutes.
8. Serve and enjoy.

Nutrition Facts
Servings: 6

Amount per serving
Calories 180

% Daily Value*

Total Fat 12.6g	**16%**
Saturated Fat 3.3g	**17%**
Cholesterol 13mg	**4%**
Sodium 155mg	**7%**
Total Carbohydrate 13.5g	**5%**
Dietary Fiber 4.8g	**17%**
Total Sugars 3.3g	
Protein 6.7g	
Vitamin D 0mcg	0%
Calcium 51mg	4%
Iron 2mg	9%
Potassium 521mg	

Roasted Cauliflower Hummus

PREP TIME: 10 Minutes

COOK TIME: 45 Minutes

SERVINGS: 12

Ingredients:

- 4 cups cauliflower florets
- 1 tsp cumin
- ¼ tsp paprika
- 1 tsp cinnamon
- 1 lemon (juiced)
- 2 tbsp maple syrup
- 2 whole garlic cloves (minced)
- 4 tbsp extra virgin olive oil
- 1 tsp sea salt
- 4 tbsp water
- ½ cup sesame seed paste

Directions:

1. Preheat oven to 200°C.
2. Grease a baking sheet with non stick spray. Set aside.
3. Place the cauliflower in a large bowl and sprinkle with 2 tablespoons of olive oil. Stir until all the florets are coated with olive oil.
4. Arrange the cauliflower into the baking sheet in a single layer. Check to ensure that the florets are not stacked on each other.

5. Place the baking sheet in the preheated oven and bake for about 35 to 40 minutes or until the cauliflower florets are tender and browned.
6. After the baking cycle remove the baking sheet from the oven and toss the cauliflower into a blender.
7. Add the sesame seed paste, salt, garlic, cinnamon, paprika and cumin.
8. Pour in the water, lemon juice and 2 tablespoons of olive oil.
9. Add the maple syrup.
10. Blend the ingredients until smooth, stopping to scrape the sides of the blender often while blending.
11. If the hummus is too thick, add more water and blend. Repeat this until you achieve your desired texture.
12. Serve the hummus into bowls and consume.

Nutrition Facts
Servings: 12

Amount per serving
Calories 95

% Daily Value*

Total Fat 7.8g — 10%
　Saturated Fat 1.1g — 5%
Cholesterol 0mg — 0%
Sodium 168mg — 7%
Total Carbohydrate 6.3g — 2%
　Dietary Fiber 1.8g — 7%
　Total Sugars 2.9g
Protein 1.9g

Vitamin D 0mcg — 0%
Calcium 74mg — 6%
Iron 1mg — 7%
Potassium 150mg

Keto Carrot Cake

PREP TIME: 15 minutes

COOK TIME: 30 minutes

SERVINGS: 20

Ingredients:

- 5 large eggs (at room temperature)
- ½ cup coconut flour
- 1 ¾ cup almond flour
- 2 tsp ground cinnamon
- 1 ¼ cups shredded carrots
- 1 ½ tsp pure vanilla extract
- ¾ cup sugar
- ¾ cup butter (melted)
- ½ cup unsweetened shredded coconut
- 2 tsp gluten free baking powder
- 1 cup chopped pecan
  Frosting:
- 8 ounce cream cheese (softened)
- ½ cup butter (softened)
- 1 tsp vanilla extract
- 1/3 cup heavy cream
- ½ cup sugar

Directions:

For the cake

1. Preheat the oven to 175°C and line two 8 inch cake pans with parchment paper.

2. In a large mixing bowl, combine the almond flour, baking powder, swerve sweetener, coconut flour and cinnamon. Mix until ingredients are well combined.
3. In another large mixing bowl, whisk together the eggs and vanilla extract.
4. Add the butter and whisk until it is well incorporated.
5. Now, gently pour the dry ingredients into the egg mixture, stirring as you add. Mix until the ingredients are well combined and smooth.
6. Fold in the shredded carrots, shredded coconut and chopped pecans.
7. Pour equal amounts of the batter into the prepared cake pans.
8. Place the cake pans in the preheated oven and bake for about 30-35 minutes.
9. After the baking cycle, remove the cakes from the oven and transfer them to a wire rack. Let the cakes sit for about 10 minutes to cool.

For the cream cheese:

10. Combine the sweetener, cream cheese, butter, heavy whipping cream and vanilla extract. Blend until smooth and fluffy. Set aside.

To assemble the layered cake:

11. Place one of the cakes on a tray and spread ½ of the cream cheese frosting over it with a knife.
12. Place the second cake over the first one and spread the remaining cream cheese frosting over it.
13. Place the carrot cake in a refrigerator and refrigerate for about 30 minutes.
14. Cut into desired sizes and serve.

Nutrition Facts
Servings: 20

Amount per serving
Calories 340

% Daily Value*

Total Fat 28.1g **36%**

Saturated Fat 12.5g **62%**

Cholesterol 92mg **31%**

Sodium 95mg **4%**

Total Carbohydrate 19.4g **7%**

Dietary Fiber 3.5g **12%**

Total Sugars 13.7g

Protein 5.9g

Vitamin D 5mcg 27%

Calcium 84mg 6%

Iron 1mg 6%

Potassium 85mg

Simple Roasted Butternut Squash

PREP TIME: 15 minutes

COOK TIME: 25 minutes

SERVINGS: 8

Ingredients:

- 1 (2 pounds) butternut squash
- 2 tablespoon extra virgin oil
- 1 tsp Italian seasoning
- ¼ tsp ground black pepper
- ½ tsp garlic
- ½ tsp cinnamon
- ¼ tsp salt

Directions:

1. Preheat the oven to 400°F.
2. Peel the butternut squash.
3. Cut the butternut squash into two (cut length wise).
4. Use a spoon to scoop out the seeds.
5. Cut the butternut squash into small chunks and wash the chunks with water.
6. In a big bowl, combine the salt cinnamon, garlic, Italian seasoning, pepper and olive oil.
7. Add the butternut squash cubes and toss until they are coated with the ingredients.
8. Line a baking sheet with foil and spread the coated chunks on the sheet.
9. Place the sheet into the oven and bake for 25 minutes.
10. Bring out the baked butternut squash.
11. Serve.

Note: If you don't want to consume the butternut snacks immediately, leave it to cool and store in a tightly sealed container

Nutrition Facts

Servings: 8

Amount per serving

Calories 55

% Daily Value*

Total Fat 3.7g	**5%**
Saturated Fat 0.5g	**3%**
Cholesterol 0mg	**0%**
Sodium 76mg	**3%**
Total Carbohydrate 6.2g	**2%**
Dietary Fiber 1.9g	**7%**
Total Sugars 1.2g	
Protein 0.5g	
Vitamin D 0mcg	0%
Calcium 4mg	0%
Iron 2mg	11%
Potassium 164mg	

Blueberry Cookies

PREP TIME: 30 minutes

COOK TIME: 10 minutes

SERVINGS: 48 cookies

Ingredients:

- 1 cup fresh blueberries
- 1 cup margarine
- ¼ tsp salt
- 2cups all-purpose flour
- ¾ tsp Ener-G baking powder (or any other renal friendly sodium free baking powder)
- 1 egg (beaten)
- 1 tsp cinnamon powder
- 1 cup white sugar
- 1 tsp vanilla extract

Directions:

1. Preheat the oven to 400°F and line a baking sheet with parchment paper.
2. Sift the all-purpose flour and baking soda into a large mixing bowl. Add cinnamon and salt. Mix until well combined.
3. In another mixing bowl, whisk together the sugar and margarine until smooth.
4. Whisk together the egg and vanilla extract in another mixing bowl.

5. Now pour the margarine mixture and the egg mixture into the flour mixture, mixing as you add the wet mixtures.
6. Mix until you form smooth dough.
7. Use a spatula to fold in the blueberries. Fold gently in other not to break the blueberries.
8. Scoop out 1 tbsp of the dough and roll into balls. Repeat until you have all the dough rolled into balls.
9. Arrange the balls into the baking sheet in a single layer.
10. Use the bottom of a glass cup to press the dough balls into flat cookies. Grease the bottom of the glass before pressing.
11. Place the baking sheet in the preheated oven and bake for 8 minutes or until the cookies are browned.
12. After the baking cycle, transfer the cookies to a wire rack to cool.
13. Serve and enjoy.

Nutrition Facts
Servings: 48

Amount per serving
Calories 72

% Daily Value*

Total Fat 3.9g	5%
Saturated Fat 0.7g	3%
Cholesterol 3mg	1%
Sodium 57mg	2%
Total Carbohydrate 8.7g	3%
Dietary Fiber 0.2g	1%
Total Sugars 4.5g	
Protein 0.7g	
Vitamin D 0mcg	2%
Calcium 18mg	1%
Iron 0mg	2%
Potassium 11mg	

Macaroni Salad

PREP TIME: 15 minutes

COOK TIME: 8 minutes

SERVINGS: 8

Ingredients:

- 1 tsp dry mustard
- ½ tsp paprika
- ½ tsp ground black pepper
- 3 cups macaroni
- ½ cup pimentos (chopped)
- 3 hard boiled eggs (sliced)
- ½ cup chopped sweet onion
- ½ cup mayonnaise
- ½ cup celery
- I small cucumber (peeled and diced)
- ½ cup grated carrot
- ½ cup chopped green pepper

Directions:

1. Bring a large pot of water to a boil and add little salt. Add the macaroni and cook for about 8 minutes or until it is tender.
2. Remove the pot from heat and rinse the cooked macaroni under cold water. Drain and set aside.
3. In a large mixing bowl, mayonnaise, carrot, pimentos, onion, cucumber, celery, sliced eggs and mustard.
4. Add the boiled macaroni and toss until the ingredients are well combined.

5. Sprinkle with pepper and paprika.
6. Cover the mixing bowl, place it in the refrigerator and chill for up to 4 hours.
7. Serve and enjoy.

Nutrition Facts Servings: 8	
Amount per serving	
Calories	**216**
	% Daily Value*
Total Fat 7.3g	**9%**
Saturated Fat 1.3g	7%
Cholesterol 65mg	**22%**
Sodium 141mg	**6%**
Total Carbohydrate 31.2g	**11%**
Dietary Fiber 2g	7%
Total Sugars 3.8g	
Protein 7g	
Vitamin D 6mcg	29%
Calcium 34mg	3%
Iron 2mg	9%
Potassium 229mg	

Crispy Pork Belly

PREP TIME: 10 minutes

COOK TIME: 6 hour 5 minutes

SERVINGS: 6

Ingredients:

- ½ pound skinless whole pork belly
- 1/3 tsp salt
- ½ tsp smoked paprika
- ½ tsp chili powder
- 1 tsp ground black pepper
- ¼ tsp onion powder

Directions:

1. Preheat the oven to 190°F.
2. Season the pork belly with salt, pepper, onion powder, and paprika. Ensure you rub the seasoning all over the pork belly.
3. Now, wrap the seasoned pork belly in parchment paper.
4. Wrap it in another aluminum foil for the second time.
5. Wrap it again with another sheet of aluminum foil for the third time.
6. Place the wrapped pork belly in a baking sheet and place the baking sheet into the preheated oven.
7. Bake for about 6 hour or until tender.
8. Remove the baking sheet and leave the wrapped pork to cool.
9. Place the wrapped pork in a refrigerator and refrigerate for about 8 hours.
10. Remove the pork belly from the refrigerator and unwrap.

11. Some fat will be dripping off the pork as you unwrap. Collect the fat with a small bowl.
12. Cut the pork belly into 6 equal sizes.
13. Now, place a large skillet on medium heat and add 2 tablespoons of the pork fat.
14. Once the fat is hot, arrange the pork belly pieces into the skillet (fat side down).
15. Sear for about 10 minutes or until the pork pieces is browned and crispy on both sides. Flip the pork pieces after the first 5 minutes.
16. Serve into plate, season with pepper and drizzle with some of the remaining pork fat.
17. Enjoy.

Nutrition Facts
Servings: 6

Amount per serving
Calories 96

% **Daily Value***

Total Fat 5.6g **7%**
 Saturated Fat 2g **10%**
Cholesterol 31mg **10%**
Sodium 153mg **7%**
Total Carbohydrate 0.5g **0%**
 Dietary Fiber 0.3g **1%**
 Total Sugars 0.1g
Protein 10.4g

Vitamin D 0mcg 0%
Calcium 10mg 1%
Iron 1mg 3%
Potassium 168mg

Cinnamon Protein Balls

PREP TIME: 45 Minutes

SERVINGS: 20 balls

Ingredients:

- 1 ½ cup creamy peanut butter (unsalted)
- ½ tsp salt
- ¼ cup sugar
- 1 tsp vanilla extract
- 2 tsp ground cinnamon
- 2 cups almond flour

Directions:

1. In a large mixing bowl, combine the almond flour, vanilla extract, cinnamon, sugar, salt and butter. Stir until the ingredients are evenly combined and the mixture is smooth.
2. Place the mixing bowl in a refrigerator and refrigerate for the mixture for about 30 minutes.
3. Remove the bowl from the refrigerator.
4. Use your hand to mold the mixture into 20 balls. You can use a spoon to measure out equal amount of the mixture to ensure that the balls are equal.
5. Serve and enjoy.
6. Store leftovers in an airtight container.

Nutrition Facts
Servings: 20

Amount per serving
Calories 195

% Daily Value*

Total Fat 14.6g	19%
Saturated Fat 2.2g	11%
Cholesterol 0mg	0%
Sodium 58mg	3%
Total Carbohydrate 9.3g	3%
Dietary Fiber 2.5g	9%
Total Sugars 4.1g	
Protein 7.8g	
Vitamin D 0mcg	0%
Calcium 28mg	2%
Iron 3mg	16%
Potassium 1mg	

Cream Cheese Cookies

PREP TIME: 15 minutes

COOK TIME: 15 minutes

SERVINGS: 15 cookies

Ingredients:

- ½ cup all purpose flour
- ½ tsp Ener-G baking powder (or any other renal friendly sodium free baking powder)
- 1/3 cup sugar
- 1 egg
- 1 tsp ginger powder
- 1 tsp vanilla extract
- ½ tsp cinnamon
- ½ cup butter (softened)
- 3 tbsp cream cheese (softened)

Directions:

1. In a medium mixing bowl, combine the butter, cream cheese and sugar
2. Add the vanilla extract and egg. Whisk until ingredients are evenly combined.
3. Mix in the flour, ginger powder, salt, baking powder and cinnamon. Mix until smooth and sticky.
4. Place to large sheet of parchment paper on a flat surface.
5. Place the dough in the middle of the parchment paper and work it into 1 cm thick flat dough with a rolling pin.

6. Roll the dough line a sausage and wrap it with parchment paper.
7. Place it in the refrigerator and refrigerate for about 1 hour.
8. Meanwhile, preheat the oven to 180°C.
9. Remove the dough from the fridge and cut into 15 round cookie using a cookie cutter.
10. Line a cookie sheet with parchment paper and arrange the dough pieces into the baking sheet in a single layer.
11. Place the cookie sheet in the preheated oven and bake until the cookies turn golden brown. This will take about 15 minutes.
12. Remove the baking sheet from the oven and leave the cookies to cool for a few minutes.
13. Serve.

Nutrition Facts
Servings: 15

Amount per serving
Calories 99

% Daily Value*

Total Fat 7.2g — 9%

    Saturated Fat 4.4g — 22%

Cholesterol 29mg — 10%

Sodium 54mg — 2%

Total Carbohydrate 7.9g — 3%

    Dietary Fiber 0.2g — 1%

    Total Sugars 4.5g

Protein 1g

Vitamin D 5mcg — 26%

Calcium 39mg — 3%

Iron 0mg — 2%

Potassium 15mg

Cinnamon Vanilla Shortbread

PREP TIME: 20 minutes

COOK TIME: 20 minutes

SERVINGS: 16

Ingredients:

- 2 tsp cinnamon
- ½ cup unsalted butter (softened)
- 1 large egg (beaten)
- ¼ tsp salt
- 2 cups all-purpose flour
- ¼ cup sugar
- 1 tsp vanilla extract

Directions:

1. Preheat the oven 150°C.
2. Line a cookie sheet with parchment paper.
3. In a large bowl, combine the cinnamon, all-purpose flour, sugar and salt. Mix thoroughly to combine.
4. In another mixing bowl, whisk the egg, vanilla extract and softened butter together.
5. Pour the egg mixture into the flour mixture and mix until the mixture forms a smooth batter.
6. Use a tablespoon to measure out equal amounts of the mixture and roll into balls.
7. Arrange the balls into the cookie sheet in a single layer.
8. Now, use the flat bottom of a clean glass cup to press each ball into a flat round cookie. Grease the bottom of the cup before using it to press the balls.

9. Place the cookie sheet in the preheated oven and bake until browned. This will take about 20 to 25 minutes.
10. After the baking cycle, remove the cookie sheet form the oven and let the shortbreads cool for a few minutes.
11. Serve and enjoy.

Nutrition Facts
Servings: 16

Amount per serving
Calories 128

% Daily Value*

Total Fat 6.4g — 8%

   Saturated Fat 0.1g — 1%

Cholesterol 12mg — 4%

Sodium 40mg — 2%

Total Carbohydrate 15.3g — 6%

   Dietary Fiber 0.6g — 2%

   Total Sugars 3.2g

Protein 2.1g

Vitamin D 1mcg — 6%

Calcium 7mg — 1%

Iron 1mg — 5%

Potassium 23mg

Chocolate Mug Cake

PREP TIME: 3 minutes

COOK TIME: 1 minute

SERVINGS: 1

Ingredients:

- ½ tsp vanilla extract
- 1 tsp olive oil
- 1 tbsp almond milk
- 2 tbsp almond flour
- 1 ½ tbsp sugar
- 2 tbsp cocoa powder
- ¼ tsp gluten free baking powder
- A pinch of salt

Directions:

1. In a small bowl, combine the cocoa powder, salt, baking powder and flour. Stir until the ingredients are all mixed and fluffy.
2. Add the vanilla, olive oil and milk. Stir until the mixture is smooth.
3. Now, pour the mixed ingredients into a mug.
4. Place the mug in a microwave and bake for 30-35 minutes on high heat.

5. Remove the cake from the oven and leave it to cool for 4 to 5 minutes.

6. Sprinkle some powder sugar on the cake and serve.

Nutrition Facts Servings: 1	
Amount per serving	
Calories	**276**
	% Daily Value*
Total Fat 16.7g	**21%**
Saturated Fat 5.2g	**26%**
Cholesterol 0mg	**0%**
Sodium 160mg	**7%**
Total Carbohydrate 34.3g	**12%**
Dietary Fiber 5.1g	**18%**
Total Sugars 25.5g	
Protein 5.3g	
Vitamin D 0mcg	0%
Calcium 295mg	23%
Iron 3mg	15%
Potassium 314mg	

Tapioca Pudding

PREP TIME: 10 minutes

COOK TIME: 15 minutes

SERVINGS: 6

Ingredients:

- 2 eggs (beaten)
- 3 cups whole milk
- ½ tsp vanilla extract
- ¼ tsp salt
- ½ cup tapioca
- ½ cup white sugar

Directions:

1. Combine the tapioca, milk, sugar and salt in a saucepan over medium to heat.
2. Bring to a boil, stirring constantly. Reduce the heat and cook for 5 minutes, stirring constantly.
3. Stir in the eggs and cook for 1 more minutes, stirring constantly.
4. Remove from heat and stir in the vanilla.
5. Serve hot or chilled.

Nutrition Facts

Servings: 6

Amount per serving

Calories 203

% Daily Value*

Total Fat 5.4g	7%
Saturated Fat 2.7g	14%
Cholesterol 67mg	22%
Sodium 166mg	7%
Total Carbohydrate 33.6g	12%
Dietary Fiber 0.1g	0%
Total Sugars 23.7g	
Protein 5.8g	
Vitamin D 54mcg	270%
Calcium 148mg	11%
Iron 1mg	3%
Potassium 196mg	

Black Bean Chocolate Brownies

PREP TIME: 10 Minutes

COOK TIME: 35 Minutes

CHILLING TIME: 12 hours

SERVINGS: 16

Ingredients:

- 1 ¼ cups sugar free chocolate chips
- ¾ cup sugar
- 1 can unsalted black beans (drained and rinsed)
- 1 tsp instant coffee
- ½ tsp Ener-G baking powder (or any other renal friendly sodium free baking powder)
- ¼ cup dark chocolate
- ½ tsp salt
- 1 tsp vanilla extract
- 3 tbsp unsalted butter (softened)
- ¼ tsp cinnamon
- 3 eggs

Directions:

1. Preheat the oven to 350°F.
2. Pat the black bean dry with paper towel and pour it into a powerful food processor.
3. Blend until the black bean is smooth.
4. Add the eggs, cinnamon, chocolate chips, dark chocolate, baking powder, salt, vanilla extract, coffee and swerve sweetener.
5. Process until smooth.

6. Line a 8 by 8 baking pan with parchment paper and pour the mixture into the baking pan. Use a spoon to smoothen and level the surface of the batter.
7. Place the baking dish in the oven and bake for about 35 minutes or until a toothpick inserted in the middle of the brownies comes out clean.
8. After the baking cycle, remove the baking pan.
9. Transfer the brownies to a wire rack to cool. Let it sit for about 10 minutes.
10. Cut into 16 equal pieces (2" by 2" square pieces).
11. Put the brownies in a fridge and refrigerate for about 12 hours for a better taste (optional)
12. Serve and enjoy.

Nutrition Facts
Servings: 16

Amount per serving
Calories 177

% Daily Value*

Total Fat 7g	**9%**
Saturated Fat 3.1g	**15%**
Cholesterol 37mg	**12%**
Sodium 144mg	**6%**
Total Carbohydrate 26.9g	**10%**
Dietary Fiber 2.6g	**9%**
Total Sugars 11.2g	
Protein 4.3g	
Vitamin D 4mcg	22%
Calcium 18mg	1%
Iron 1mg	5%
Potassium 117mg	

www.ingramcontent.com/pod-product-compliance
Lightning Source LLC
Chambersburg PA
CBHW030943240526
45463CB00016B/1448